DATE DUE

5/5/99	
MAY - 4 1999	
MAY - 2 2007	

GAYLORD   PRINTED IN U.S.A.

Treating Alcoholism and Drug Abuse Among Homeless Men and Women: Nine Community Demonstration Grants

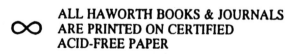

Treating Alcoholism and Drug Abuse Among Homeless Men and Women: Nine Community Demonstration Grants

Milton Argeriou, PhD
Dennis McCarty, PhD
Editors

Preparation of this volume was supported by grant 1 R18 AA07915 from the National Institute on Alcohol Abuse and Alcoholism

The Haworth Press
New York • London

Treating Alcoholism and Drug Abuse Among Homeless Men and Women: Nine Community Demonstration Grants has also been published as *Alcoholism Treatment Quarterly*, Volume 7, Number 1 1990.

The Haworth Press, Inc., 10 Alice Street, Binghamton, NY 13904-1580
EUROSPAN/Haworth, 3 Henrietta Street, London WC2E 8LU England

Library of Congress Cataloging-in-Publication Data

Treating alcoholism and drug abuse among homeless men and women : nine community demonstration grants / Milton Argeriou, Dennis McCarty, guest editors.
    p.   cm.
    "Also published as Alcoholism treatment quarterly, vol. 7, no. 1, 1990"--T.p. verso.
    Includes bibliographical references.
    ISBN 0-86656-992-8 (alk. paper)
    1. Homeless persons—United States—Alcohol use—Case studies. 2. Homeless persons—United States—Drug use—Case studies. 3. Alcoholics—Rehabilitation—United States—Case studies. 4. Narcotics addicts—Rehabilitation—United States—Case studies. 5. Alcoholism—Treatment—United States—Case studies. 6. Drug abuse—Treatment—United States—Case studies. I. Argeriou, Milton. II. McCarty, Dennis, Ph.D.
HV5140.T74   1990
362.29'18'086942–dc20   90-4301
                                                CIP

Treating Alcoholism and Drug Abuse Among Homeless Men and Women: Nine Community Demonstration Grants

CONTENTS

ABOUT THE EDITORS

Milton Argeriou, PhD, has been involved in the field of substance abuse since 1969. His efforts have been divided among the areas of research, evaluation, and program administration. Dr. Argeriou is currently Project Director of the Stabilization Services Project, one of the nine NIAAA Community Demonstration Projects for Homeless Substance Abusers. He has worked on several other national demonstration projects, most notably, the Alcohol Safety Action Projects funded by the Department of Transportation. Dr. Argeriou was also co-founder of Alcohol and Health Research Services, a non-profit corporation dedicated to conducting substance abuse research and program evaluation that has been and continues to be a major element in the development of substance abuse policy and programming in the State of Massachusetts. His publications have appeared in the major alcoholism journals.

Dennis McCarty, PhD, has primarily been interested in the evaluation of alcoholism and drug abuse treatment, intervention, and prevention services. He is currently Director of Policy and Evaluation for the Massachusetts Department of Public Health, Division of Substance Abuse Services, which develops addiction treatment services and alcohol and drug-free housing for homeless adults and families. Dr. McCarty is also the Principal Investigator for the Stabilization Services Project, an NIAAA community demonstration grant that develops and evaluates shelter-based programs for alcoholism and drug abuse treatment.

Nine Demonstration Grants: Nine Approaches

Dennis McCarty, PhD

Street life for homeless men and women abusing drugs and/or alcohol can be confusing, dangerous, and frustrating. Individuals shuffle unsteadily between detoxification centers, shelters, bus stations, subways, day programs, jail, abandoned buildings, and soup kitchens. It is a painful life complicated by, but also made more bearable because of the use and abuse of alcohol. Homeless individuals impaired as a result of abusing alcohol or other drugs may require multiple types of service in an integrated continuum of care. Ideally, care begins in detoxification and extends through stabilization services and placement in relatively permanent housing. Case management may be used to enhance engagement and retention in care. Almost every review of services for the homeless, however, stresses the need to demonstrate, evaluate, and compare different interventions and systematically assess effectiveness (Baumhol, 1987; Morrissey & Dennis, 1986; Mulkern & Spence, 1984; Rog et al., 1987; Wittman, 1985).

Section 613 of the Stewart B. McKinney Homeless Assistance Act (Public Law 100-71) authorized the National Institute on Alcohol Abuse and Alcoholism, in consultation with the National Institute on Drug Abuse, to fund community demonstration grants to develop and expand alcohol and drug abuse treatment services for homeless men and women. Nine grants were awarded. Programs are located in Alaska (Anchorage), California (Los Angeles and Oakland), Kentucky (Louisville), Massachusetts (Boston), Minnesota (Minneapolis), New York, (New York City), and Pennsylvania (two projects in Philadelphia). The programs represent a broad spectrum of engagement, intervention, and recovery approaches and focus on a range of primary client characteristics. Major pro-

1

gram services and significant client features are summarized in Table 1. Programs are identified by the city. The Philadelphia programs are differentiated by the applicant agency—Diagnostic and Rehabilitation Center (DRC) and Horizon House. While programs share many features, they also reflect the unique needs and opportunities in each community. An overview of the similarities and differences sets the context for the project chapters. Four issues are reviewed: clients, project services, project implementation, and evaluation.

CLIENTS

The homeless are not limited to older, white, male alcoholics. Currently, men and women who are homeless or at risk of homelessness are a heterogeneous population. They are young and old, people of color, women and children, mentally ill, and are likely to abuse drugs in addition to alcohol. The demonstration projects, therefore, serve a range of clients. Women receive services in seven programs. Two programs (New York and Philadelphia/DRC) serve only women. In Oakland, about 40% of the participants are women. Women in Anchorage, Boston, Los Angeles, and Philadelphia/Horizon House reflect their presence in the target population—10% to 20%. Louisville and Minneapolis are limited to men.

Large proportions of the clients in Anchorage (60%) and Minneapolis (58%) are Alaskan Natives or American Indians. Other projects serve substantial numbers of Black (Boston, Los Angeles, Louisville, New York, Oakland, and both Philadelphia sites) or Hispanic (Los Angeles, New York, and Philadelphia/DRC) clients.

Homeless individuals with mental illness require special services. The Philadelphia/Horizon House project specifically targets its engagement and rehabilitation services toward the homeless suffering from both mental illness and alcohol and drug abuse. Anchorage and Boston also report that significant proportions of their clients have dual diagnoses.

A final characteristic is the use of alcohol and drugs. In general, clients report using both drugs and alcohol. Older chronic inebriates, however, are more likely to use alcohol more heavily or exclusively. Minneapolis limits services to chronic public inebriates (individuals with 15 or more prior detoxifications) and Anchorage, Boston, Louisville, Los Angeles and Oakland expect to serve many chronic alcoholics with histories of frequent detoxifications. Younger clients report more variety in their drug of choice and are more likely to use both drugs and alcohol or use drugs exclusively, primarily cocaine (including crack) and heroin. The Philadelphia DRC project works primarily with cocaine dependent women and their children. Similarly the New York and Oakland projects report a high incidence of crack use among the women and children they serve. The Boston project serves both alcoholics and drug addicts. While most participants (90%) report drinking alcohol, over half (56%) of the Boston participants also report a drug problem and 20% report a primary addiction to heroin or cocaine.

PROJECT SERVICES

Project services and approaches vary widely. Differences are both philosophical and programmatic. The two California programs, for example, provide services for individual clients but tend to emphasize environmental and systemic change as an effective tool for fostering community wide reductions in alcohol and other drug-related problems. The other sites recognize the value of environmental and systems modification but stress services to individuals. Minneapolis also articulates a clear message of controlling access to services to foster more effective use of appropriate resources and reducing the large costs of medical, legal, and social services associated with many chronic public inebriates.

Programmatic differences tend to be driven more by community needs and target populations than project philosophy. The major components are outreach, sobering-up stations, residential services, housing, and case management.

The three programs that work primarily with women (New York, Philadelphia/DRC, and Oakland) emphasize outreach services to build trust and to encourage service utilization. Drop-in centers and day programs are important in the New York and Oakland sites. The Philadelphia/Horizon House project for the dually diagnosed also emphasizes engagement and the development of therapeutic relationships. Louisville provides a jail liaison both as an outreach

TABLE 1. Major Client Characteristics and Program Components in the Nine Community Demonstration Grants

Characteristic/Service	Anchorage	Boston	Los Angeles
SPECIAL CLIENT CHARACTERISTICS			
Women	0	0	0
Chronic Inebriates	0	0	0
Drug Addicts		0	
Dual Diagnosis	X	0	
American Indian/Alaskan Native	X		
Blacks/Latinos		0	0
SERVICES			
Outreach/Engagement			
Jail Liaison			
Drop-in Center/Day Program	X		
Sobering-up Station	X		
Detoxification	X		
Post-detox Stabilization		X	X
Recovery Home/Residential	X	0	X
Sober Housing	X	X	X
Outpatient			
Case Management		X	
Medical Services			
Vocational Services		0	0

X = Primary Service or Client Characteristic
0 = Service Available or Clients Included
   ᵃOakland program includes the indicated services. Individuals may enter at any point and need not move from one level to the next. Emphasis is on the service system.

Louisville	Minneapolis	New York	Oakland[a]	Philadelphia/ DRC	Philadelphia/ Horizon
		X	X	X	0
X	X		X		
0		0	0	X	
	0				X
	X				
0		0	0	0	0
	0	X	X	0	X
X	0				
		X	X		
X			X		
	0			X	0
					0
			X	X	X
	X	X	X		
	0	0		X	X
X	X				X
	0		X	X	0
X	0	X		X	0

mechanism and as a strategy to reduce the costs associated with arrests for public intoxication.

Sobering-up stations and reception centers are key project components in Anchorage, Louisville, and Oakland. In Anchorage and Louisville, clients use the service as a safe place to sleep off inebriation. Staff encourage entry to formal detoxification and recovery programs. Post-detoxification residential services vary from a short but variable length ($M = 35$ days) stabilization services in Boston to longer-term services in Philadelphia. The Stabilization Services in Boston provide a safe environment to continue post-detoxification physical and cognitive recuperation while waiting for a placement in a recovery home or therapeutic community. Los Angeles uses a 90-day post-detoxification service to prepare clients for a more demanding residential service that reintegrates the participant into the community. In Oakland, residential lengths of stay were shortened and services intensified so that system capacity could be increased and services provided to more homeless. Finally, the Philadelphia/DRC project has developed a longer-term residential program for women and children.

The development of alcohol and drug-free housing is emphasized in all project cities. Each program recognizes that the greatest need among the homeless is a safe place to live. For individuals with alcohol and drug problems, safety requires a sober environment. While sober housing may not be available for each project participant, each project attempts to foster alcohol and drug-free living environments. Some sites use subsidies and loans to encourage housing.

Case management is a project component in five sites. The approaches to case management reflect a variety of strategies. Minneapolis adopted a specific model that has demonstrated success among clients who are mentally ill. Philadelphia's Horizon House works with dually diagnosed clients but uses a different approach to case management. Louisville and Boston both emphasize client empowerment and benefit acquisition but have not adopted explicit orientations. Louisville uses case management to encourage clients to detoxify and enter treatment. Boston, on the other hand, does not start case management until clients near the completion of stabilization and enter recovery homes. Comparisons among these approaches may help articulate a clearer philosophy to case management with alcoholics and drug addicts.

IMPLEMENTATION

During the first year projects struggled to varying degrees with implementation. Projects relate key implementation issues in their chapters. One issue that might otherwise be overlooked is the structure of the project sponsor. Five of the projects are nonprofit social service agencies (Anchorage, Louisville, New York, and both Philadelphia sites). The other four projects' sponsors were either county (Los Angeles, Minneapolis, Oakland) or state alcohol/drug (Boston) authorities. The nature of implementation problems varied. Anchorage, Philadelphia/DRC and Philadelphia/Horizon House struggled with community or owner resistance to siting programs in specific locations. New York changed project sites because of changes in city policies with respect to "welfare hotels." The county authorities have struggled more with contracting (Oakland), staffing (Minneapolis), and staff resistance to new services (Los Angeles). The political entities were less likely to try to site and establish new services and more likely to build on existing services.

EVALUATION

As Community Demonstration sites, each project is committed to documenting implementation and services and assessing outcomes. Replication in other communities necessitates a clear history of process and effects. NIAAA required all projects to dedicate 25% of their resources toward process and outcome evaluation and collaborate with the national evaluation effort.

The local evaluation designs illustrate the application of many experimental and quasi-experimental approaches to the assessment of outcome. One study cannot provide a definitive statement on the best services for the homeless. The variety of services and evaluation approaches, included in the national demonstrations, however, will permit a clarification of the services that may be more effective for discreet subgroups of clients. Gradually, a more complete mosaic of data and programmatic experience will develop and lead providers and policy makers toward more complete answers.

The nine grants have begun the process of identifying effective recovery approaches for homeless men and women with alcohol and drug problems. Documentation and dissemination of the results and process starts with this volume. NIAAA and the nine projects collaborated and developed this joint record of project descriptions and reviews of the first year of implementation. Each project has prepared a separate chapter. The first chapter provides an overview of NIAAA's efforts with the homeless, the national evaluation and a discussion of major observations from year one. Successive chapters review each project. Projects are organized alphabetically by city.

ACKNOWLEDGMENTS

The editors and chapter authors thank those who have made the projects possible. First, we are deeply grateful to the men and women struggling with addiction who participate in the projects and through their successes and failures become pioneers easing the way of those who follow. Secondly, the outreach workers, case managers, counselors, housing managers, and demonstration staff provide the structure, glue, and human touch that programs require for success; without their deep commitment to serving the homeless, there would be no programs. Finally, we thank the leadership at NIAAA for their continued concern and commitment to the issue of homelessness and for supporting the demonstration programs. NIAAA's Homeless Demonstration Branch (Barbara Lubran, Robert Heubner, Janet Ruck, and special consultant Gerry Garrett) and Grants Management Branch (Elsie Flemming) have motivated and encouraged us during implementation. The staff, subcontractors, and consultants from R.O.W. Sciences (Scott Crosse, Howard Goldman, Susan Ridgely, and Nancy Smith) and C.L.E.W. Associates (Fried Wittman and Patricia Shane) have provided consultation, guidance, and technical assistance to each project and coordinated the national evaluation. We appreciate the assistance we have received from everyone and look forward to our second and third years.

REFERENCES

Baumhol, J. (1987). *Research Agenda: The Homeless Population With Alcohol Problems*. Rockville, MD: NIAAA.

Morrissey, J. P. & Dennis, D. L. (1986). *NIMH-Funded Research Concerning Homeless Mentally Ill Persons: Implications for Policy and Practice*. Bethesda, MD: NIMH.

Mulkern, V. & Spence, R. (1984). *Alcohol Abuse/Alcoholism Among Homeless Persons: A Review of the Literature*. Rockville, MD: NIAAA.

Rog, D. J., Andronovich, G. D., & Rosenblum, S. (1987). *Intensive Case Management for Persons Who are Homeless and Mentally Ill*. Washington, DC: Cosmos Corporation.
Wittman, F. D. (1985). *The Homeless with Alcohol-Related Problems*. Proceedings of a meeting to provide research recommendations to NIAAA. Rockville, MD: NIAAA.

Alcohol and Drug Abuse Among the Homeless Population: A National Response

Barbara Lubran, MPH

During the past decade, the characteristics of the homeless population in the United States have changed significantly. Once considered the plight of the stereotypical skid row alcoholic, the homeless population now includes increasing numbers of women, children, the elderly, minorities, the unemployed, runaway teenagers, displaced families, and the mentally ill. Estimates of the size of the homeless population range from 250,000 (HUD, 1984) to as many as 3 million (Hombs and Snyder, 1982). A recent HUD survey of shelters for homeless individuals estimates that the daily occupancy of homeless shelters is approximately 180,000 persons (HUD, 1989). In addition to being without stable shelter, these individuals tend to face multiple problems including poverty, malnutrition, unemployment, physical and mental illness, isolation, and alcohol and/or other drug problems (Institute of Medicine, 1988).

An extensive body of literature exists on the history of homelessness, the demographic and social characteristics of the homeless, and trends relating to homelessness. Study findings show that the growing homeless population is becoming more diverse. These trends are attributed to changes in the economy, a decline in low income housing units, and reductions in social entitlements and related services (Institute of Medicine, 1988; Garrett, 1989). Although studies describe the magnitude and characteristics of the

Barbara Lubran is Director, Homeless Initiative, National Institute on Alcohol Abuse and Alcoholism, Parklawn Building, Room 16C-02, 5600 Fishers Lane, Rockville, MD 20857.

homeless population in general, little is known about what interventions, treatment approaches, and combinations of services are most successful in addressing the problems faced by homeless individuals (Interagency Council on the Homeless, 1988).

Among the many interrelated factors contributing to the increasing numbers of homeless individuals, alcohol remains most significant. Recent studies suggest that about 35 percent of homeless adults have alcohol problems (HUD, 1989; Fischer and Breakey, 1987; Garrett and Schutt, 1986; Koegel and Burnam, 1987; Wright and Knight, 1987). In addition, estimates of the number of homeless individuals with drug problems range from 10 percent (Millburn, 1989) to 25 percent (HUD, 1989). Further compounding the problem, homeless persons who drink heavily are susceptible to health problems, such as trauma, gastrointestinal disorders, thermoregulatory disorders, vascular disorders, infestations, and tuberculosis (Wright and Knight, 1987).

Legislative Action

In July 1987, Congress passed the Stewart B. McKinney Homeless Assistance Act (Public Law 100.77) "to provide urgently needed assistance to protect and improve the lives and safety of the homeless." The first comprehensive Federal initiative aimed at helping this country's homeless population, the McKinney Act addresses the needs of homeless persons in the areas of emergency food and shelter, health and mental health care, housing, educational programs, job training, and other community services. Section 613 of the Act specifically authorizes funds for the National Institute on Alcohol Abuse and Alcoholism (NIAAA) in consultation with the National Institute on Drug Abuse (NIDA) to establish a demonstration program for homeless persons with alcohol and/or other drug problems.

This article provides a review of the NIAAA Community Demonstration Grant Projects for Alcohol and Drug Abuse Treatment of Homeless Individuals. It covers the history and design of the program, challenges faced, the treatment demonstration models, evaluation efforts, initial findings, and implications for future policy and programming efforts.

NIAAA HOMELESS INITIATIVES

Since 1984 NIAAA has supported a variety of initiatives designed to help generate research and to document and disseminate research findings concerning programs for homeless individuals with alcohol problems. Activities in this area include: developing a literature review on alcohol problems among the homeless population; convening an expert panel resulting in recommendations to the Institute on research priorities for this area; and sponsoring a research conference on "Homelessness, Alcohol and Other Drugs." NIAAA has also encouraged researchers to study the role of alcohol in conjunction with other drug and mental health problems among the homeless population (i.e., those with dual diagnoses and multiple service needs).

A NATIONAL DEMONSTRATION PROGRAM

Responding to the legislative mandate for the establishment and funding of new Federal programs serving the homeless population, NIAAA, in consultation with NIDA, launched the first nationwide Federally-funded demonstration program focusing on treatment and recovery approaches to address the complex issue of alcohol and other drug problems among the homeless population. In the Fall of 1987, NIAAA issued a Request for Applications for Community Demonstration Grant Projects for Alcohol and Drug Abuse Treatment of Homeless Individuals, a program designed to provide grants for demonstration projects that develop, expand, and evaluate alcohol and other drug treatment and recovery services for homeless individuals. This program represents the first NIAAA-supported demonstration effort in eight years. The tremendous demand for this type of demonstration is evidenced by the number of community-based organizations that responded to the request for grant applications. Eighty-eight applications were received in response to the request. A Special Peer Review Committee met in the Spring of 1987 to judge the applications. Based on the level of available funding, nine grants with the best priority scores were funded in Fiscal Year 1988 for a two year period.

Program Goals

The goals of the Community Demonstration Grant Projects for Alcohol and Drug Abuse Treatment of Homeless Individuals are to provide, document, and evaluate successful and replicable approaches to community-based alcohol and/or other drug abuse treatment and rehabilitation services for individuals with alcohol and/or drug related problems who are homeless or at imminent risk of becoming homeless. The program goals are designed to (a) decrease levels of alcohol and/or other drug use, (b) increase cooperation and formal linkages among alcohol treatment, drug treatment, and other supportive services in addressing the special needs of this population with alcohol and/or drug related problems, (c) improve access to shelter and housing (including alcohol and drug-free living environments), (d) increase health and mental health status, (e) enhance economic status, and (f) improve quality of life.

It estimated that during the first two years of funding, more than 16,000 homeless individuals will receive some services from the nine demonstration projects. It is further estimated that over 20% of all individuals served will receive an intensive level of treatment and/or services (NIAAA, 1988).

Program Considerations

In designing this national demonstration program, NIAAA recognized the many challenges facing programs in their efforts to respond to the needs of homeless individuals with alcohol and/or other drug-related problems.

- Existing alcohol and drug treatment programs and services do not adequately respond to the needs of the target population. There is tremendous difficulty in providing services to clients who do not have fixed residences. They present unique challenges for outreach, tracking, treatment, and follow-up efforts (DHHS, 1987).
- Treatment approaches must address multiple, interrelated needs (i.e., alcohol and/or drug treatment, housing, health care services, employment services, etc.). A homeless person who is an alcohol and/or other drug abuser is unlikely to bene-

fit from an approach that does not include a full range of services (Institute of Medicine, 1988).

- Few agencies have the capacity to address the homeless person's interrelated needs for treatment/recovery services, housing, health services, and employment services. Better coordination and cooperation among service delivery systems in the community is required. One method for systems coordination is a case management approach which involves assigning responsibility to a person or, to the extent possible, a team of persons to maintain a long-term, supportive relationship with the client, regardless of where the client is and regardless of the number of service agencies involved.

- Community-based agencies serving the target population seldom have the research capability required to evaluate their efforts, thereby limiting future replication efforts. Evaluation is a vehicle through which more can be learned about which approaches work best with which clients under what conditions. Information from program evaluations can help improve the operations of existing programs and inform future policies for addressing the multiple needs of the homeless population.

PROGRAM INFORMATION AND PRODUCTS

NIAAA has supported a number of efforts designed to promote information exchange and dissemination among the demonstration projects, researchers, service providers, policymakers, and others in the field. In May 1988, NIAAA developed a *Synopses of Community Demonstration Grant Projects for Alcohol and Drug Abuse Treatment of Homeless Individuals*. This report describes the programs participating in the demonstration; their goals and objectives, services, and target populations; and planned activities.

In October, 1988, NIAAA developed *Alcohol and Other Drug Abuse Among Homeless Individuals: An Annotated Bibliography*. This document presents state-of-the-art literature in three topic areas: (1) the prevalence of alcohol and other drug abuse among homeless individuals; (2) treatment and service approaches for homeless populations with alcohol, drug, and dual disorder problems; and (3) evaluation methodology and instrumentation with regard to measurement of the primary and secondary objectives of the demonstration.

In order to provide a uniform taxonomy for collecting and reporting data on the activities of the demonstration projects and other organizations related to homeless individuals with alcohol and/or other drug problems, NIAAA developed *Services for Homeless People with Alcohol and Other Drug Problems: A Taxonomy for Reporting Data on the Utilization of Services and on Systems Level Linkage Activities*. This document provides standard definitions related to treatment activities, and activities intended to develop linkages between organizations concerned with the homeless population.

In February 1989, NIAAA sponsored a research conference on "Homelessness, Alcohol and Other Drugs" at the University of California at San Diego (supported through a grant to the Alcohol Research Group of the Medical Research Institute of San Francisco). The conference provided the opportunity for researchers and service providers to share findings and strategies for working with the homeless population with alcohol and/or other drug problems. A report containing proceedings from the conference is available through the National Clearinghouse on Alcohol and Drug Information.

These and future information dissemination activities will be part of NIAAA's ongoing program to transmit information derived from research and demonstration projects to health care providers, program administrations, State and local officials, researchers, educators, and others in the field.

TREATMENT DEMONSTRATION MODELS

The NIAAA Community Demonstration Grant projects are located in eight cities: Anchorage, Alaska; Boston, Massachusetts; Los Angeles, California; Louisville, Kentucky; Minneapolis, Minnesota; New York, New York; Oakland, California; and two projects in Philadelphia, Pennsylvania.

Eight of the projects (Boston, Minneapolis, Los Angeles, Anchorage, Louisville, New York and the two projects in Philadelphia) are conducting client outcome studies with comparison groups; the Oakland project evaluation uses a pre-test and post-test design without a comparison group to assess client outcomes. Anchorage and the Horizon House project in Philadelphia are evaluating services targeted at the dually-diagnosed population (i.e., those individuals with mental illness and concomitant alcohol and/or other drug problems). The New York project is demonstrating a comprehensive outreach/intervention service for homeless women with children residing in SRO (single room occupant) hotels. The Diagnostic Rehabilitation Center project in Philadelphia is evaluating treatment services for homeless mothers and their children. Native Americans and Native Alaskans comprise a large proportion of the target population for both the Minneapolis and the Anchorage projects.

Several of the projects utilize intensive case management techniques to support the client's functioning in the community. Outreach – in the shelters, welfare hotels, or on the streets – is a process used by several of the projects to engage clients. Other unique components within the demonstration projects include a jail liaison program, vocational education, and housing assistance. The long-term recovery needs of homeless alcoholics is addressed through job-training programs and, ultimately, long-term alcohol-free housing. Various opportunities for housing assistance exist in many of the programs and range from long-term alcohol-free living environments to boarding homes and low demand residences.

PROGRAM EVALUATION

Based on NIAAA's recognition of the challenges in implementing the demonstration programs and desire to enhance the ability to measure the success and replicability of these programs, the national demonstration program plan emphasizes evaluation research. Given the dearth of information on successful services for the target population, the evaluation component is particularly important in this demonstration program. In order to ensure that grantees placed a priority on the evaluation research, 25% of each grant award was earmarked for evaluation purposes. Programs were encouraged to establish formal linkages with local universities or other organizations that could provide the required research expertise. In order to measure the success and replicability of the demonstration programs, evaluations will be conducted at both the project level and on a national level, to the extent possible, across all sites.

The individual project process level evaluations will describe program activities and clients; and assess the attainment of program objectives.

The national evaluation is designed to address several key questions about the implementation of the nine demonstration projects: the level and types of services provided, characteristics of clients, and program effects. The national evaluation will also attempt to determine which models/methods work and which don't work for different homeless populations and why. The information used to address these questions will be contributed by the individual project evaluations. The project evaluations are the building blocks of the national evaluation. The role of the national evaluation is to increase comparability among projects on data and research (e.g., by requesting the use of some common instruments); assist the projects to conduct evaluations and provide data for the national evaluation; present information from the projects in a standardized format; conduct secondary analyses on project data as appropriate; and synthesize information across projects with similar interventions and clients as appropriate. The national evaluation will also assess the extent to which positive program effects can be replicated in other settings.

Through the national evaluation, it may be possible to determine which individuals were effectively reached, served, and treated using different methods and approaches. The evaluation results will be used to facilitate replication of successful services for treating alcohol and/or other drug problems in the homeless population and as a basis for further research.

INITIAL FINDINGS

A number of interim process findings have emerged from the NIAAA Homeless Demonstration program and an analysis of the challenges the demonstration programs confronted during the early stages of program development and implementation. Although these findings do not represent the definitive research findings from the demonstration projects, they may have implications for the design of future programs and services to address the problem of alcohol and/or other drug abuse among the homeless population.

- Many of the program applicants recognized that the traditional treatment/recovery approaches are not effective, in and of themselves, with homeless individuals with alcohol and/or other drug problems because these approaches don't go far enough in facilitating reentry into the community. Based on this experience, more socially-oriented recovery approaches are being applied (i.e., alcohol-free living centers, case management, etc.).
- There is general agreement that continuity of care is essential. This indicates the need for and importance of case management, follow-up, and aftercare services. For many demonstration programs, case management is a critical program component. Because of the complexity of the problems/needs presented, it is important to refer clients to, and help them utilize, a variety of services within and outside the community.
- Because of the length of time required to institute a change in existing systems and structures, it has been difficult for the homeless demonstration projects to operationalize a systems change approach. Systems-change is a lengthy process, therefore, it is important that systems change efforts continue in conjunction with service delivery. Preconceptions about the target population and programs traditionally designed to serve homeless people resulted in projects facing considerable community opposition during program implementation. Commonly referred to as the "NIMBY" phenomenon (Not In My Back Yard), there was resistance to both the population being served and the new service methods. An active citizens advisory board is one vehicle being used to reduce community resistance.
- The programs discovered that there was a tremendous demand for their services. There was a significant unmet need for services for homeless individuals with alcohol and/or other drug problems who had been excluded or turned away from other

service systems, including traditional homeless projects. Alcohol and drug treatment programs have also been reluctant to serve the homeless because many are unpredictable, cause trouble, present medical problems and risks, and make extreme demands on service providers.

- Two major barriers to program start-up were encountered: facilities acquisition and renovation, and staffing.
- Community resistance, zoning restrictions, and the need for renovations caused unanticipated frustrations and delays. Horizon House in Philadelphia reported that "Although we had the resources to purchase a building . . . , we were unable to locate one for purchase that was suitable . . . Instead, we had to choose to lease a building with an option to buy. As a result, with far less control over construction than if we were directly contracting for renovations, we found ourselves facing delays in completion of the facility." The complex problems presented by the homeless population make it difficult to recruit and retain the type of staff needed for projects of this type. Staff dropout rates are typically very high and staff burnout tends to be an ongoing problem.
- Because the demonstration programs developed their own research designs independently, as part of the grant application process, it was more difficult to structure the national evaluation than NIAAA originally anticipated. This problem emerged from the need to obtain the level of standardization required for the national evaluation. Because the collaboration process was initiated after the initial project start-up phase, compromises needed to be made to achieve a level of standardization.

IMPLICATIONS FOR FUTURE EFFORTS

Despite gaps in our current knowledge, there are programmatic implications for the demonstration program. The implications include suggestions for treatment/recovery methods, program design strategies, future research studies, and Federal policies related to the problems of the homeless population with alcohol and/or other drug problems.

More Clearly Defined Service Interventions

Demonstration projects (of the type described in this chapter) are designed to test new, innovative, and improved ways (i.e., models, approaches, methods, techniques) of reaching and delivering services to target populations. These projects provide an opportunity to test and evaluate service interventions and methods that hold promise of being successful in other settings. To be successful, demonstration projects must be adequately structured and the interventions applied (i.e., services, methodologies) must be clearly and adequately defined.

Interventions That Build Upon What Has Been Learned

To understand and learn how to effectively address emerging social problems (such as homelessness), it is useful to design, conduct, and evaluate demonstration projects. Such demonstration efforts make it possible for researchers and program planners to: (a) learn how to best reach target populations, (b) pool data and information to assess and understand target groups, (c) test and compare methods and approaches across sites, (d) determine which subjects do better or worse in different service settings, and (e) share knowledge. Demonstrations provide flexibility in the implementation phase. Investigators can adjust and alter strategies and approaches, based on what is learned. By evaluating approaches tried by the demonstration projects, the field will be able to advance to new designs and prepare rigorous research studies of the most promising approaches.

Standardization of Research and Evaluation

It is difficult to conduct experimental studies, particularly when researchers do not have easy access to study populations (such as the homeless), do not possess enough knowledge about the population at risk, and cannot control for all of the variables. It is particularly challenging to conduct controlled studies that involve homeless individuals because they are difficult to reach at follow-up. Therefore, in organizing a collaborative demonstration project involving grant programs (each responsible for their own independent studies), it is important to establish the framework for research standardization as early as possible. Once programs establish individualized questionnaires and research tools, it becomes increasingly difficult to achieve standardization in the demographic, clinical, and service data being collected.

Planning Sufficient Time
for Program Implementation

Through the process evaluation, which is part of the NIAAA demonstration program, the causes for delays in program start-up and the different elements that impact on programs during the implementation phase, are being documented. Adequate time is needed in initiating a demonstration program, creating new service systems for homeless populations with alcohol and/or other drug problems, and developing the research methodology and tools required to evaluate results and outcomes.

REFERENCES

Fischer, P.J. and Breakey, W.R. (1987) Profile of the Baltimore homeless with alcohol problems. Alcohol Health and Research World, 11(3):36-41.

Garrett, G. (1989) Once over lightly: An historical overview of research on alcohol problems and homelessness. National Conference on Homelessness, Alcohol and Other Drugs, San Diego, CA, February 2-4.

Garrett, G.R. and Schutt, R.K. (1986) Homeless in the 1980s: Social services for a changing population. Presented at the Annual Meeting of the Eastern Sociological Society, New York City.

Hombs, M.E. and Snyder M. (1982) Homelessness in America: A forced march to nowhere. Washington, D.C.: Community for Creative Nonviolence.

Institute of Medicine. (1988) Homelessness, Health, and Human Needs. National Academy Press.

Interagency Council on the Homeless. (1988) A Nation Concerned: A Report to the President and the Congress On the Response to Homelessness in America. Washington, D.C.

Koegel, P. and Burnam, M.A. (1987) Traditional and non-traditional homeless alcoholics: Alcohol Health and Research World, 11(3):28-32.

Millburn, N. (1989) Drug abuse among the homeless. In J. Momeni (editor), Homeless in the United States (Vol.II), Westport, CT: Greenwood Press.

U.S. Department of Health and Human Services. (1987) Alcohol Health and Research World, Homelessness, 11(3):3.

U.S. Department of Housing and Urban Development. (1984) A Report to the Secretary on the Homeless and Emergency Shelters, Washington, D.C.
U.S. Department of Housing and Urban Development. (1989) A Report on the 1988 National Survey of Shelters for the Homeless, Washington, D.C.
Wright, J.D. and Knight, J.W. (1987) Alcohol Abuse in the National "Health Care for the Homeless" Client Population: A Report to the National Institute on Alcohol Abuse and Alcoholism. Social and Demographic Research Institute, University of Massachusetts, Amherst.

Treating Homeless and Mentally Ill Substance Abusers in Alaska

Raymond A. Dexter, EdD

Clitheroe Center is a comprehensive substance abuse treatment program operated by the Salvation Army in Anchorage, Alaska. It is the largest of such agencies in the State and has been in operation since October, 1976. Prior to the receipt of the current NIAAA Homeless Demonstration grant, the Agency included a Community Service Patrol (a basic life support ambulance service to transport inebriates to homes, hospitals or other treatment facilities), a 20 bed modified medical detoxification center, a 38 bed residential treatment facility, a specialized women's residential facility for 12 adults and 4 pre-school children, a 12 bed half-way house and an extensive outpatient facility. The Salvation Army also operates Eagle Crest, an alcohol free living center or "dry hotel" as part of their constellation of services in the Anchorage area. The demonstration grant utilizes all these services to expand the capability to serve homeless substance abusers.

Anchorage, as the regional hub for Southern and Western Alaska, has developed a sizable homeless population estimated at slightly in excess of 4,000 individuals. The majority is in the 20-40 year old range with about half of them classified as alcohol abusers and 300 to 400 as chronically mentally ill. Because of the severe Alaskan winters, one critical need targeted by the Municipality of Anchorage was to provide some kind of shelter where inebriated people could be provided sobering services. Other shelters for the homeless refuse to admit intoxicated individuals, and hypothermia cases are common admissions to local hospitals.

Raymond A. Dexter is affiliated with The Salvation Army, Clitheroe Center, P.O. Box 190567, Anchorage, AL 99519-0567.

Since a sizable number of homeless substance abusers are also diagnosed as mentally ill, it seemed appropriate to team up with the local mental health center, Southcentral Counseling Center, to provide services to this population. Accordingly, the NIAAA grant was designed to include a Diagnostic Screening Center, a walk-in counseling and sobering service in the core area of Anchorage. Another focus of the grant was to provide joint substance abuse and mental health treatment to those referred from the screening center into treatment.

PROJECT IMPLEMENTATION

After receipt of the NIAAA grant, a psychiatrist was hired and assigned to Clitheroe Center to conduct evaluations and a weekly group with dual diagnosed clients. An outpatient counselor from the Clitheroe Center conducted weekly group and individual counseling sessions at the mental health Transitional Living Center.

Securing a facility for the Diagnostic Screening Center was not easily achieved. About 90 percent of the owners of buildings in the target area refused to rent their buildings for this program. Part of the problem was the initial cost of bringing the building up to institutional occupancy code. A few owners simply didn't want to be associated with such a program. A building was finally secured and permits requested through the Planning and Zoning Commission. A three month wait followed until the public hearing. During this time, Project Leadership addressed the local Community Council, spoke to neighboring businesses (it was a fringe area with many vacant stores, a tattoo parlor, an "X rated" night club as well as more respectable establishments), and secured letters of support from a variety of sources. However, it was clear that trouble was coming when the president of the bank that was located across the street from the proposed site called and said he'd have to cancel his letter of support. Several of his larger depositors had threatened to withdraw their deposits if he went on record as supporting this program.

When the time for the public hearing arrived, a few witnesses had been assembled who testified about having operated such a shelter in other communities, about the need for a shelter in Anchorage, about the traffic patterns of street people, and a variety of other rational arguments for establishing the service in the selected site. The opponents of the project painted a vivid picture of inebriates being brought in from all over the city and dumped on the doorsteps of the shelter neighbors. For three successive weeks, the Commission was regaled with horror stories of unspeakable acts which could be anticipated should the shelter be established. Emotion won out over reason and the Commission denied the permit.

Soon afterwards, another site was located which was still farther away from the businesses that had led the previous opposition. However, the new site didn't even get to the permit request stage. The businessman who owned the building was threatened with a boycott if he leased the building to the Project. He withdrew his offer and the Project was back to the beginning again. By this time, the first snows had fallen, and the newspapers and television stations had become heavily involved in supporting the project and the mayor had proclaimed a health alert to expedite the location and use of a facility as a shelter. The tide of public opinion had swung in favor of the homeless. The owner of Artic Camp and Equipment donated four modular units left over from the Alaska pipeline construction camps. Alyeska Pipeline Services Company provided transport vehicles to move the units down from the Yukon River, to a site donated by the Municipality of Anchorage. The Alaska Chapter of the National Fire Sprinklers Association donated and installed the sprinkler system. Employees from the Municipality Health and Human Services and Property and Facilities Management Departments, and volunteer carpenters, electricians and laborers from local unions all contributed their services in an effort to complete the building before the intense cold of January.

The modular structure has become the temporary shelter and screening center for the project. In the meantime, the Municipal Health and Social Services Commission conducted hearings regarding the location of the permanent facility. Their recommendations have been approved by the Municipal Assembly and the way is now clear for the facility to be located in the general area originally selected, without further public hearings. As a further demonstration of support, the City is now negotiating for the purchase of a building and the State Office of Alcohol and Drug Abuse has agreed to provide funds to do the necessary remodeling for code compliance and program design.

PROJECT OPERATION

The Diagnostic Screening Center, even in its temporary form and location, has become the vital first link in the treatment of the homeless substance abusers. The staff at the Center has been recruited chiefly from former homeless people who have completed treatment at the Clitheroe Center and have achieved an extended period (2 years) of sobriety. We have found that they have been able to establish rapport with the clientele at the Center and to instill hope for a better way of life. There have been a few instances in which the recovering counselors have discovered that their rather tenuous sobriety was threatened by the constant flow of inebriated persons through the center. This has been, and will continue to be a concern of our clinical staff and is always addressed in the weekly staff meetings as well as in individual sessions.

When the Screening Center staff is successful in motivating clients into treatment, the first stage is usually the Clitheroe detoxification unit at Point Woronzof. After detox, clients enter the extended care residential program located in the same facility. The program is approximately 70 days in duration and is designed specifically for homeless chronic substance abusers. It includes much slower paced educational classes on alcohol and other substances of abuse, AA and NA step groups, growth groups to identify personal goals and work on behaviors identified as dysfunctional, weekly individual counseling sessions, and physical, social, cultural and recreational activities to aid clients address all facets of daily living. A heavy emphasis is placed on vocational education. This includes a vocational assessment focusing on employment-seeking skills, job retention skills, employment history, relevant interests, aptitudes, attitude and values, physical and mental limitations, resources and supports, aspirations, and knowledge of the job market. The vocational program offers a wide range of vocational support services, with career counseling, testing, development of job seeking skills and employment and educational referrals.

Almost a third of the homeless experience chronic mental illness. An initial diagnosis is done by a psychiatric nurse and a mental health clinician meets with this sub-group on a weekly basis. Experience has shown that quite often latent mental illness is masked by the effects of the substances abused until about one month of treatment has elapsed. A thorough psychiatric evaluation is done on clients believed to be mentally ill unless they have come into the program with a confirmed DSM III R diagnosis.

Once a diagnosis has been established, this sub-group of the treatment population receives weekly individual and group counseling by a treatment team composed of both substance abuse and mental health clinicians. Prescribed medication is administered by Clitheroe Center nursing staff. Weekly interdisciplinary case conferences monitor the progress of clients through treatment.

After the residential phase, clients are referred to the Clitheroe Center Transitional Care Unit or to the Transitional Living Center operated by the Community Mental Health Center. Some, able to make it on their own, are referred to Eagle Crest, the alcohol free living center maintained by the Salvation Army. In all cases, continued treatment is maintained by the counseling staff at the Clitheroe Center Outpatient Component.

PROGRAM ASSESSMENT

In the first five months of the program over a thousand (N = 1,097) different individuals utilized the Diagnostic and Screening Center for more than 10,000 admissions. While this number is almost double the expected goal for the entire first year, the characteristics of the population have remained essentially as expected. The clients are 84% male, 60% are between 25 years and 44 years of age, and 60% are Alaska natives.

Assessment of program effectiveness is based on intergroup comparisons of clients who complete treatment, clients who drop out of treatment, and clients who were screened only. Data collected at screening, during treatment, and at intervals following treatment are used to assess treatment outcomes. The data include: demographic data, drinking and drug taking behavior, social and psychological functioning, economic and occupational information and criminal behavior. Data analyses will provide insight into factors that may lead to successful treatment of this population which has been historically resistant to traditional kinds of treatment.

Stabilization Services for Homeless Alcoholics and Drug Addicts

Dennis McCarty, PhD
Milton Argeriou, PhD
Milly Krakow, PhD
Kevin Mulvey, PhD

Boston's strong regional economy, rapidly escalating housing costs, and the depletion of rental units through conversion to condominiums have contributed to the development of a substantial homeless population. A one night census suggested that approximately 3,000 homeless men and women were sleeping in shelters, the streets, the airport, bus stations and abandoned buildings throughout Boston ("Recent City Census," 1986).

In 1983, Governor Dukakis made homelessness his major human service initiative. Beginning with a "Profile of the Homeless in Massachusetts" (Kaufman & Harris, 1983), the administration crafted and successfully passed the nation's first comprehensive legislation directed toward homelessness (M.G.L. Chapter 450, Acts of 1983). The Act removed the need to have an address to be eligible for state entitlement benefits such as AFDC, General Relief, and Food Stamps. Emergency assistance was provided for families in need of shelter and permitted advances for rent and security deposits. The Administration has subsequently sponsored, and

Dennis McCarty is affiliated with the Division of Substance Abuse Services, Massachusetts Department of Public Health, 150 Tremont Street, Boston, MA 02111. Milton Argeriou and Kevin Mulvey are affiliated with the Stabilization Project, 200 Lincoln Street, Boston, MA 02111. Milly Krakow is affiliated with Health & Addiction Research, Inc., 867 Boylston Street, Boston, MA 02116.

passed, legislation to control condominium conversions and to provide funding for low and moderate income housing. The "Massachusetts Comprehensive Policy Approach to Homelessness" (Johnston, Kaufman, & Anthony, 1987) continues to guide service development.

Substance Abuse

Alcohol and drug abuse often complicate the lives of homeless men and women. The proportion of homeless in Boston who also have substance abuse problems is consistent with national studies and ranges between 29 and 52 percent for men and 7 to 16 percent for women (Schutt & Garrett, 1985, 1986; Bassuk, Rubin, & Lauriat, 1984, 1986). Approximately one-quarter have both alcohol and mental health problems. An analysis of admissions to alcohol detoxification centers in Boston found that one-half of the admissions were homeless (38%) or at risk of homelessness (11%). The homeless and at risk homeless were predominately male (89%), and white (77%). They were older ($M = 45$ years) than non-homeless clients ($M = 40$ years) and less likely to be working (6% vs 27%).

Service Gaps and Needs

Massachusetts and Boston provide a wide array of innovative services for the homeless (Rog, Andronovich, & Rosenblum, 1987; Wittman & Madden, 1988). Both the Governor and the Mayor are committed to reaching out to the homeless and finding ways to stabilize their difficult lives. Most who work with the homeless feel that Boston has a variety of important services in place. The integration of services, however, could be stronger. Alcoholics and drug abusers who are homeless frequently lack the motivation or skill to seek out currently available services. Even when sober, admission and utilization procedures can be complicated. For newly detoxified individuals who are in early recovery and often are still struggling with physical weakness and impaired cognitive functioning, the tasks are nearly impossible. Increased stabilization services, coupled with case management, therefore, were suggested as ways to increase service coordination.

Stabilization

Any one detoxification is unlikely to lead to sobriety (Finn, 1985). A study of 447 clients admitted to detoxification centers in Massachusetts during a seven month period counted 1,023 detoxification admissions (McCarty, Mulligan, & Argeriou, 1987). Finn (1985) suggested that services for public inebriates would improve with longer stabilization and "drying out" periods and improved interagency coordination. Clients would benefit from more time off the streets and coordination would enhance the likelihood of moving to the next level in the continuum of care. Cognitive functioning in long-term alcoholics is impaired to the point that a three to five day detox is inadequate for physical and cognitive recuperation and the chronic inebriate may be unable to engage in anything but the most basic treatment programs. This may be one reason chronic alcoholics do so poorly in recovery homes when referred directly from detoxification and provides a rationale for a transitional care experience geared directly for chronic, homeless alcoholics and drug abusers (Gubar & Reading, 1978).

Case Management

The homeless often distrust service providers and institutions because of real or imagined poor treatment in the past or the difficulty in negotiating the bureaucratic system to access the services they need (Breakey, 1987). Disaffiliation, mobility, and multiplicity of needs hinder the homeless alcoholics access to services. Services are often fragmented, with little coordination and integration between agencies. In projects with both alcoholics (Neuner & Shultz, 1986) and with mentally ill patients (Rog et al., 1987), case managers demonstrated ability to overcome the distrust of clients, coordinate treatment and life support needs, and successfully stabilize the chronically homeless.

PROJECT DESCRIPTION

The Stabilization Services Project provides post detoxification services to substance abusers in Boston, Massachusetts who are homeless or near homeless. Continued substance abuse treatment through placement in recovery homes, transitioning to residence in sober housing and a resumption of employment are the major elements of the planned post stabilization rehabilitation. In addition, half of the Project participants receive case management services to assist them along the continuum.

Stabilization services are provided at four sites: two in substance abuse treatment agencies – Boston Detox Transitional Care Facility and STAIR (Short-term Addiction Intervention Residence); and two in community based shelters for the homeless – Long Island Shelter and Shattuck Shelter. Each site has 10 beds dedicated to clients in the demonstration project. Clients remain for as long as it takes to achieve a recovery home placement. The mean length of stay across all four sites for all clients is 22 days. However, some clients stay as long as 60 or more days before a placement is made. Figure 1 provides an operational schematic of the Project.

Project Entry

Project entry occurs through detoxification centers in the Boston area. All potential candidates must be detoxified and meet 10 criteria: (1) medically clear and in reasonable good health, (2) homeless or at risk for homelessness, (3) eighteen years of age or older, (4) presence of a substance abuse problem, (5) stable mental health, (6) willing to participate and be randomly assigned to placement, (7) no prior admissions to the demonstration project, (8) not currently enrolled in another program or treatment, (9) not currently employed and (10) no on-going criminal justice system involvements/court dates.

Candidates are usually screened every weekday. When beds are available at any of the four sites, the entry points are called in a predetermined random order to identify potential program participants. All participating detoxification centers have an equal chance of placing clients in the project. Accepted clients are randomly assigned to available beds by the evaluation director. Clients are transported to the stabilization sites by detoxification center personnel.

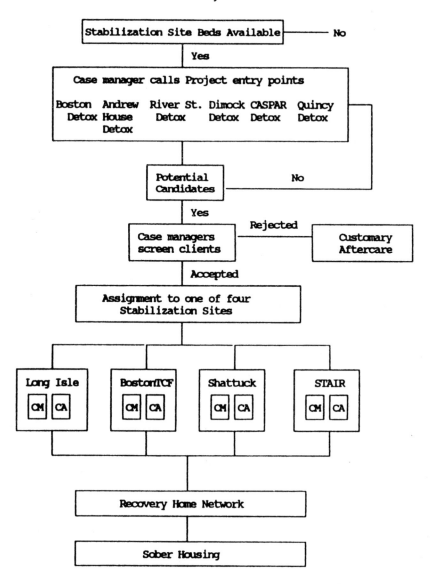

FIGURE 1. Stabilization Services Project Daily Selection and Service Procedures

Stabilization Services

Stabilization services are provided in treatment programs and in shelters. Services in treatment programs tend to be more structured, have less free time, and provide a greater assurance of an alcohol and drug free environment.

Boston Detox Transitional Care Facility

The 40-bed Transitional Care Program at Boston Detoxification Center gives newly sober men and women additional time to continue recuperation. Eight male and two female beds are dedicated to Stabilization Services Project clients. Services are based on a five-point program philosophy: (1) a client's life is unlikely to improve without assistance, (2) idleness encourages passive dependent behaviors and does not challenge the behaviors that contribute to homelessness and substance abuse, (3) new and healthier behavior patterns must be introduced and practiced actively, (4) future orientation increases the client's personal investment in behavior change, and (5) supportive reality therapy clarifies client focus and goals. Group counseling and daily self-help (AA and NA) meetings are required. Since opening in 1982, the program has evolved and become more structured.

Short-Term Addiction Intervention Residence (STAIR)

STAIR is a 40-bed program serving homeless and near homeless men and women with alcohol and/or drug problems. STAIR opened in 1984 to provide an alcohol and drug-free environment in which substance abuse treatment and treatment planning could occur. Most STAIR clients have struggled with alcoholism and/or drug abuse for a long time with unsuccessful attempts at recovery. They are unemployed, homeless, and alienated from society. STAIR also works, however, with clients who are new to treatment. The Stabilization Project reserves eight beds for men and two for women.

STAIR is the most structured program. The intensive residential substance abuse treatment includes evaluation and treatment planning, individual and group counseling, identification of health care needs with referral to appropriate medical care. Substance abuse education and health education are integral parts of the programming along with AA and NA participation. STAIR encourages residents to view treatment from a consumer perspective. Clients interview residential programs and seek the service that is best for them, not necessarily the program with the first available bed.

Long Island Shelter

The Long Island Shelter for the Homeless is located on an island in the middle of Boston Harbor on the grounds of Long Island Chronic Care Hospital. Since opening in 1983, Long Island Shelter has expanded several times and currently serves 420 persons each night. There is a strong service philosophy. An intake clinic orientates each guest to shelter procedures and a Nursing Clinic takes a medical history for each guest.

Individual and group counseling and AA and NA participation constitutes the core of the stabilization services provided and accounts for most of the daily programming. Physical and social activities rebuild individuals in both areas. The program is limited to 10 beds for men. Because alcohol and drug use is difficult to prevent among other shelter guests, the Stabilization Unit is a substance abuse treatment program operating in a "wet" setting. Consequently, the maintenance of sobriety is difficult. The physical separation of the ten stabilization beds in an attractive private room contributes to the maintenance of sobriety and appears to help to bond stabilization clients to each other, give them a sense of identity and generate mutual support for the maintenance of their sobriety.

Shattuck Shelter

The Shattuck Shelter for the Homeless is a 170 bed (200 bed winter capacity) shelter serving homeless adults with overnight care, food, and clothing. A comprehensive health care and social services program is provided for the guests. Services include (a) a 24-hour medical respite for homeless individuals recovering from illnesses or injuries, (b) a transitional program for the working homeless, (c) veterans' counseling for substance abusers, (d) elderly case management and placement services, and (e) Alcoholics Anonymous meetings.

Stabilization Services Project programming at the Shattuck Shelter is similar to the Long Island Shelter programming. Individual and group counseling, AA and NA group meetings, alcohol and health education and recreation are the basic elements of the Shattuck program. Expressive therapy is also available. A full-time site coordinator manages the Stabilization Project within the Shelter. The site coordinator is assisted by two shelter social workers who work directly with Project clients. Project clients are housed on the second floor of the Shelter with guests enrolled in the shelter's working program. The separation of Project clients helps insulate them from the larger transient substance using/abusing population of shelter guests. However, separation is not as complete as at the Long Island Shelter. Unlike the other stabilization sites, efforts to place Project clients begin immediately upon admission. As a result, the average length of stay at the Shattuck Shelter is the shortest of all four sites.

Case Management

The case manager was conceived as a travel companion rather than a travel agent (Deitchman, 1980). Case managers work to empower clients; assisting them but not doing for them what they can do for themselves. Case managers perform five basic functions: assessing needs, planning to meet needs, linking the client to services, monitoring the client's progress, and advocating for the client (Rog et al., 1987; Sullivan, 1981).

Each stabilization site has its own case manager who works collaboratively with the site coordinator or a site staff person who has been specifically assigned to the Project. Case managers are also assigned to specific detoxification centers where they screen potential clients. Detoxification liaison (4.2 hrs/week) and site liaison (4.7 hrs/week) constitute major case manager responsibilities. Together, the two activities consume almost one-quarter of the case managers' work week. Other major activities include travel (4.3 hrs/week) and networking with other agencies (3.7 hrs/week). Case managers develop rapport with all clients assigned to a stabilization site. Random assignment to case management occurs after three weeks of stabilization and the intensity of involvement increases.

Case managers help clients reach decisions regarding their recovery and guide them along the recovery continuum. Case managers are not therapists but facilitators who link clients to needed services, monitor their involvement and provide support when needed to maintain recovery. Case managers play a significant role in networking client services and developing linkages between the Project and Community agencies. Case managers serve as ambassadors of the Stabilization Services Project and work to establish the Project as a viable resource within the treatment community. Linking the Stabilization Project to the recovery home network was a primary concern at the outset of the Project. Case managers played major roles in this effort. A client referral to a particular halfway house was the basis for initiating contact, establishing a dialogue and developing a mutually acceptable plan of action for the referred client.

Linkages

The need for multiple services often evident among men and women living in shelters and on the street, requires closer linkages among agencies working with the homeless. Stabilization Services has fostered relationships and has met with more than 200 separate groups during the first year. A six session training program has been one of the most important linkage efforts. The program examined case management, alcoholism, drug abuse, mental illness, and AIDS among the homeless. There were 77 participants from 36 agencies including shelters, health centers, and substance abuse treatment services. The training sessions generated great interest and have contributed to collaboration between the Department of Public Health, the Department of Public Welfare, and the Shelter Providers Association to sponsor additional training on substance abuse and on AIDS for shelter staff.

Evaluation Design

The evaluation design compares the four demonstration stabilization services, with and without intensive case management, on processes and outcomes using multiple methods (e.g., client self-report, staff interviews, and treatment observations and records) and multiple measures (e.g., client satisfaction, client participation, reported alcohol and drug use, and days to readmission in detox). Inclusion of two examples of programs based in shelters and two based in substance abuse treatment agencies, helps differentiate effects due to specific sites or counselors from more generalizable effects that are found across settings and individuals.

Evaluation Instruments

Structured client interviews are conducted at screening, admission, discharge or 30 days (whichever comes first), and 90, 180, and 270 days post-admission. The screening assessment is used to verify that patients have recovered to the point that they are not confused or disoriented, they have no serious cognitive impairments, and they comprehend the interviewer's questions and informed consent process. Clients who pass the screening interview are assigned randomly to a demonstration service.

Within 48 hours of arriving at the assigned project, clients complete a one to two hour admission interview. The interview, conducted by the staff of the stabilization service, includes: (1) a management information system interview, (2) the 25 item Alcohol Dependence Scale (Skinner & Horn, 1984) and (3) the Addiction Severity Index (McLellan et al., 1980), and (4) a review of current living conditions.

Discharge interviews are conducted at termination or at 30 days (whichever occurs first) and include the discharge information and the Client Satisfaction Questionnaire (Larsen et al., 1979). The interview records discharge status and assesses client perceptions of the demonstration service. Client satisfaction is one indicator of the program's ability to meet client needs. Clients also rate the counselors and case managers who handle their case.

Follow-up interviews are conducted 90, 180, and 270 days post admission. The interviews monitor current living situation, employment, participation in treatment, and drug and alcohol use. The evaluation staff and case managers conduct follow-up interviews.

PRELIMINARY RESULTS

Between August 15, 1988 and June 19, 1989, 410 men and women were screened for program participation and 366 (89%) met all admission criteria and were assigned to a project site. Not all clients arrived at their assigned site. Clients were most likely to enter services at STAIR ($n = 70$, 99% of referrals), Shattuck Shelter ($n = 105$, 95% of referrals), and Long Island Shelter ($n = 77$, 94% of referrals). Boston Transitional Care had the lowest referral completion rate ($n = 82$, 80% of referrals).

The admission interviews suggest that stabilization clients have substantial alcohol and drug problems, histories of mental illness, and few social or economic resources. Program participants tended to be unmarried (never married = 64%, divorced = 19%, separated = 13%, widowed = 1%), men (88%) without a college education (high school graduate = 36%, less than high school graduate = 38%). The mean age was 35 years and one-third (31%) were veterans (WWII = 3%, Korean = 9%, Vietnam = 31%, peace time = 58%). Almost all (94%) reported a need for treatment for alcohol problems and many (65%) also requested treatment for drug problems. One-quarter (23%) reported using drugs intravenously during the year prior to admission. Over half (58%) said that they were slightly (14%), moderately (12%), considerably (13%) or extremely (19%) troubled by psychiatric problems.

Despite their histories of prior admission to alcohol (74%), drug (41%), inpatient mental health (25%) and outpatient (29%) treatment, more than half (55%) completed stabilization. Completion rates ranged from 59% (Boston Transitional Care) and 58% (Long Island Shelter) to 55% (STAIR) and 50% (Shattuck Shelter).

The mean length of stay for all discharges was more than three weeks (24 days). Clients who completed treatment had longer stays ($M = 35$ days) than those who dropped out ($M = 11$ days) or were discharged administratively ($M = 22$ days). STAIR clients required the longest time to complete their stay ($M = 47$ days) because placement efforts do not begin until clients have been in the program for three weeks. The other programs used 28 days (Shattuck), 32 days (Boston Transitional Care), and 35 days (Long Island) to place clients in longer-term residential care.

Clients are randomly assigned to case management or customary aftercare on day 21 of their stay in the stabilization program. As of June 19, 1989, 219 clients had achieved this milestone. Approximately half ($n = 113$) were assigned to customary aftercare.

Implementation Process

Stabilization and case management for homeless substance abusers have been accepted as valuable additions to available rehabilitative services. Two types of resistance to random assignment, however, have been observed: client and staff. Only a few individuals screened have refused to participate specifically because of random site assignment. Anecdotal reports suggest, however, that some potential clients refuse the screening interview because of the possibility that they may be assigned to a less preferred program. Staff resistance to random assignment was found primarily among detoxification and stabilization site personnel. Reduction of resistance was achieved by stressing the value of the demonstration project, the need for randomization and the benefits accruing to project participants regardless of where they were placed or whether they received a case manager.

A second barrier to implementation is the cooperation and collaboration between Project case managers and treatment agency staff. Treatment agency resistance to continued involvement of Project case managers disrupts client monitoring and follow-up efforts. To counteract the resistance, Project leadership and staff use a case by case approach in which treatment agencies and recovery homes are individually instructed regarding the Project. Project case managers assure treatment agency staff that the case managers will not duplicate or undermine treatment agency staff efforts. Case managers efforts are to complement and supplement, not to supplant or subvert the work of treatment agency staff. This approach has been highly successful.

Women and ethnic minorities are significant subgroups of the homeless substance abusers serviced by the Stabilization Services

Project. So far, 12% of Project clients are women, 40% are African American, and 5% are Latino. Blacks and women are somewhat over represented when compared to data from Boston area detoxification centers. At the outset of the Project, women were assigned to all four stabilization sites. Detoxification and stabilization staff, however, were concerned because female clients were housed with the general population of female shelter guests, many of whom were active substance abusers. Separate sleeping areas in the two shelter settings were available for men clients but not women participants in the Project. Women were restricted, therefore, to the two alcohol treatment agencies where all women are seeking to maintain their sobriety. The stabilization of female clients in shelter settings appears to require a separate and secure area of the shelter. The number of women in a shelter based stabilization unit also needs to be great enough to provide "strength in numbers" and an identity apart from other women in the shelter.

One of the persistent problems encountered during the early months of the Project was communication. Some of the difficulty was related to start-up and a lack of clarity in describing the project to clients and site staff. It became clear, however, that the persistence of communication difficulties, particularly among project entry staff and stabilization site personnel was due to the number of individuals involved, staff turnover and the many other responsibilities borne by these individuals. The solution was also clear, message repetition, continued project orientation sessions and staff training.

Programming needs to be coherent, organized and plentiful. Based on observations of daily activities at the stabilization sites, it has become apparent that the amount of "free time" and the level of client involvement varies across sites. To reduce diversity, a program coordinator will be added to the Project staff to assist sites and provide leadership in program development and enrichment.

DISCUSSION

In spite of multiple addictions, histories of prior treatment, noticeable levels of psychiatric problems, and a lack of social and economic resources, many clients completed stabilization. The 165 men and women remained in care for a mean of 35 days and were placed in longer-term residential treatment. Those who did not complete treatment still averaged 11 days of continued sobriety and recuperation. The preliminary results encourage our continued efforts to develop and improve alcoholism and drug abuse treatment programs for homeless men and women. Stabilization services appear to make substantial contributions to recovery among homeless men and women. It appears feasible, moreover, to provide stabilization services in treatment programs and in shelter settings.

REFERENCES

Bassuk, L., Rubin, L. & Lauriat, A. (1984). Is homelessness a mental health problem? *American Journal of Psychiatry, 141,* 1546-1548.

Bassuk, L., Rubin, L. & Lauriat, A. (1986). Characteristics of sheltered homeless families. *American Journal of Public Health, 76,* 1097-1101.

Breakey, W. R. (1987). Treating the homeless. *Alcohol Health and Research World, 11* (3), 42-46.

Deitchman, W. S. (1980). How many case managers does it take to screw in lightbulb? *Hospital and Community Psychiatry, 31,* p. 789.

Finn, P. (1985). Decriminalization of Public Drunkenness: Response of the Health Care System. *Journal of Studies on Alcohol, 46,* 7-23.

Gubar, G. & Reading, E. (1978). One Approach to the Treatment of the Skid Row Alcoholic. *Journal of Alcohol and Drug Education,* Vol. 23, No. 3, 66-76.

Johnston, P. W., Kaufman, N. K., & Anthony, A. A. (1987). The Massachusetts approach to homelessness. In *Homelessness: Critical Issues for Policy and Practice.* Boston: The Boston Foundation.

Kaufman, N. K. & Harris, J. (1983). *Profile of the Homeless in Massachusetts.* Boston: Massachusetts Executive Office of Human Services.

Larsen, D. L., Atkisson, C. C., Hargreaves, W. A., & Nguyen, T. D. (1979). Client Satisfaction Questionnaire. In D. J. Lettieri, J. E. Nelson & M. A. Sayers (Eds.), *NIAAA Treatment Handbook Series 2: Alcoholism Treatment Assessment Research Instruments.* (DHHS Publication No. ADM 85-1380). Rockville, MD: National Institute on Alcoholism and Alcohol Abuse.

McCarty, D., Mulligan, D. H., & Argeriou, M. (1987). Admission and referral patterns among alcohol detoxification patients. *Alcoholism Treatment Quarterly, 4* (1), 79-90.

McLellan, A. T., Luborsky, L., O'Brien, C. P., & Woody, G. E. (1980). An improved evaluation instrument for substance abuse patients: The Addiction Severity Index. *Journal of Nervous and Mental Disease, 168,* 26-33.

Neuner, R. P. & Schultz, D. V. (1986). *"Borrow Me A Quarter" Study.* Anoha, Minnesota: Minnesota Institute of Public Health.

Recent City Census (1986, October 12). *Boston Globe*.

Rog, D. J., Andronovich, G. D., & Rosenblum, S. (1987). *Intensive case management for persons who are homeless and mentally ill*. Washington, DC: Cosmos Corporation.

Schutt, R. K. & Garrett, G. R. (1985). *The Long Island Shelter Interview Study: Assessing Intake Procedures*, (Report to the City of Boston). Boston: Department of Health and Hospitals, University of Massachusetts at Boston.

Schutt, R. K. & Garrett, G. R. (1986). *Homeless in Boston in 1985: The View from Long Island*. Boston: Long Island Shelter Project, University of Massachusetts at Boston.

Skinner, H. A. & Horn, J. L. (1984). *Alcohol Dependence Scale User's Guide*. Toronto: Addiction Research Foundation.

Sullivan, J. P. (1981). Case management. In J. A. Talcott (ed.), *The Chronically Mentally Ill*. New York: Human Science Press.

Whittman, F. & Madden, P. (1988). *Alcohol Recovery Programs for Homeless People: A Survey of Current Programs in the U.S.* Rockville, Maryland. National Institute on Alcohol Abuse and Alcoholism.

The Sober Transitional Housing and Employment Project (STHEP): Strategies for Long-Term Sobriety, Employment and Housing

Al Wright, JD
Juana Mora, PhD
Lou Hughes, PhD

During the past two decades, programs for homeless alcoholics have generally been limited to short-term emergency shelter, detoxification, and primary alcoholism recovery services. These activities have tended to be ineffective in meeting the long-term sobriety, employment and housing needs of homeless alcoholics (Wittman, 1989).

Projects over the past several decades have often followed one of the following two models:

Skid Row Detoxification — Urban Recovery

Skid Row Detoxification — Rural Recovery

While the two models show success for short-term sobriety, such ancillary support services as intensive vocational guidance and job search activities, accessing of training opportunities and implementation of long-term planning for independent living have not been incorporated into the program designs.

The Los Angeles demonstration program established a service model for exploring the premise that "greater amounts of adjunct

Al Wright, Juana Mora, and Lou Hughes are affiliated with the Los Angeles County Office of Alcohol Programs, 714 W. Olympic Boulevard, Suite 1000, Los Angeles, CA 90015.

47

support . . . appear necessary for many homeless clients who lack the skills and habits to support an alcohol-free life-style" (Wittman, 1989:1). The target population reflects the composition of the Los Angeles County homeless population, which is disproportionately male and ethnic minorities. The chronically homeless and alcoholic men and women in the program lack sufficient work skills or work history to permit employment after departure from a primary alcohol recovery program.

The STHEP project is the first in Los Angeles County to address the long-term recovery, vocational, and housing needs of homeless alcoholics, with a comprehensive evaluation plan incorporated into the design and implementation of the project. The evaluation component documents and evaluates the service model for the purpose of informing researchers, program planners, and administrators on effective service approaches for the target population.

BACKGROUND AND STATEMENT OF THE PROBLEM

Existing services for the homeless alcoholic do not offer an effective transition from Skid-Row to non Skid-Row environments but tend to focus exclusively on short-term recovery and survival issues. For example, the Weingart Center located at Sixth and San Pedro Streets in central Los Angeles, is a ten-story social service center providing primary detoxification, emergency housing, nutrition, and health care for homeless or disadvantaged persons. The Weingart Center emphasis is on taking care of the immediate and pressing basic physical needs of individuals. Its services are designed for brief periods of time (five to thirty days), as turnover and demand for beds are high in the area.

Many of the graduates from the Weingart Center are referred to two large rural alcohol recovery centers: Warm Springs, located 50 miles northwest of Los Angeles in a wooded mountain area, and the Antelope Valley Rehabilitation Center (AVRC), located in the high desert town of Acton some 40 miles from Los Angeles. Participants reside in such programs for approximately 90 days and receive alcoholism recovery services, career counseling, basic skills instruction, and pre-employment training. As most of the residents of

Warm Springs and Acton formerly lived and worked in central Los Angeles, they usually return to the inner city. However, there are no specific programs available to assist persons with securing long-term housing and employment, nor are there services dedicated to assure a successful re-entry into independent living in an inner city community. Thus, the recidivism rate for both models (Skid Row Detoxification — Urban Recovery, and Skid Row Detoxification — Rural Recovery) remains high with estimates ranging from 70 to 80 percent (Los Angeles County Plan, 1988).

TARGET POPULATION
AND PARTICIPANT SELECTION

The target population for the STHEP program is characterized as having a history of chronic alcoholism and homelessness, an absence of marketable and employable skills and being economically and socially disadvantaged. Prospective STHEP participants were referred to the Antelope Valley Rehabilitation Center (called "Acton" after its location) during their participation in various social model detoxification programs. STHEP participants consisted of persons who agreed to participate in a seven month program (3 months at the rural Acton location and 4 months at Mary Lind, an urban alcohol recovery center in Los Angeles) with the goal of maintaining sobriety, obtaining stable employment and securing permanent housing.

PROGRAM GOALS AND SERVICES

The goals of the STHEP program are to provide alcoholism recovery, vocational rehabilitation, and housing services, and evaluate their effectiveness on homeless alcoholics in Los Angeles County.

STHEP involves a two-phase residential recovery program. Phase I consists of participation in a 90 day, 20-bed residential primary alcohol recovery and pre-employment program provided at a rural location in Acton, California. Phase II involves participation in a 120 day, 20-bed, transitional recovery, employment and housing program at an Alcohol Recovery Center of the Mary Lind Foundation, located in central Los Angeles. The program and progression of phases are designed to encourage self-sufficiency and sustained recovery among the participants. Phases I and II shift from a structured, treatment-oriented environment to a self-initiated and self-sustaining program of personal recovery which can be maintained after participants leave the project. The program provides participants with effective transition periods moving from the urban, skid-row alcohol-involved environment to a rural alcohol recovery location, then proceeding to a downtown transitional center which provides programs for sobriety, housing and job search.

Services in both Phases I and II include health, exercise, nutrition, and legal services; AA meetings; education and employment counseling; and social events.

PROGRAM SUMMARY

Phase I: Acton. Homeless alcoholics from Skid Row area of Los Angeles and currently in social model detoxification programs are referred to a rural alcohol recovery program. The first 90 day phase provides the initial recovery, pre-employment and adjunct support such as health, mental health, and educational needs of the participants. An individualized recovery and education plan is developed for each person. Services in the 90 day recovery phase include individual counseling, alcohol education, and participation in nutrition, exercise and pre-employment activities. As residents approach departure from Phase I, each participant, with assistance from Program Advocates and vocational staff, develops an exit plan which contains provisions for maintaining sobriety, stable employment, long-term housing, supportive sober social networks, and related social service needs. At departure from Phase I, residents are encouraged to join the STHEP alumni group, and to return to the facility to provide volunteer help to newly recovering people. Those persons who enter Phase I and do not complete are referred as appropriate to detoxification services, recovery programs, and housing or employment agencies as required.

Phase II: Mary Lind. Participating graduates of the Acton phase return to Los Angeles and stay at this urban alcohol recovery center for 120 days. Transitional housing, employment training, and supportive recovery services are continued in this smaller urban facility, and participants are re-introduced to the inner city environment. Services focus on preparing participants to re-enter society through development of social skills while living in a sober, supportive environment. Services include vocational training and education, job search activities, self-help recovery activities and assistance in obtaining long-term housing.

Systems Linkage. In addition to the direct recovery services offered to clients in Phases I and II, the STHEP program contains an innovative System-Level Linkage component which assists the network of alcohol agency co-service providers to ". . . develop new knowledge about the homeless with alcohol-related problems, and their treatment, housing, and support needs" (Lubran, 1987:73). The Systems Level Linkage unit provides technical assistance to alcohol agencies to increase the number of affordable housing units and employment opportunities for alcohol recovery center residents. The purpose of this additional component to STHEP was to build and strengthen the supply of housing, employment, and support services in the local community and thus assure the availability and access to such key services for STHEP graduates.

EVALUATION

The project evaluation is an integral part of the program, and is being conducted by the Prevention Research Center (PRC). Features of the evaluation include the availability of a randomized control group (Acton residents with similar profiles as STHEP participants); integration in the Office of Alcohol Program's (OAP) existing tracking and outcome data collection systems (Kline et al., 1987); a retrospective study of project completers and non-completers; and a process evaluation which studies the program environment and the program's responsiveness to participants' service needs. The following components are included in the evaluation:

- Collecting and analyzing demographic, process, and outcome data on all project participants and a control group of participants in other alcohol-related services.
- Monitoring the delivery of services to evaluate conformance to service program goals, values and objectives.
- Performing an intensive retrospective study of a sample of participants that complete and a sample that do not complete the project, including semi-structured interviews with participants and staff.
- Tracking all project participants and a sample of non-participants through the County-funded alcohol-related services system to determine patterns of service usage and outcomes.
- Evaluating the process and outcome of system-level linkage efforts among resource agencies for the homeless.
- Informing County-level policy and program development units concerning the alcohol-related problems of the homeless, and linking findings with the national database.

ADMINISTRATION

The Office of Alcohol Programs (OAP) administers, coordinates, and provides the technical and scientific direction for the project. The OAP subcontracts with the Mary Lind Foundation and the Prevention Research Center (PRC), and has developed a memorandum of understanding with the County-operated Acton program to provide project services. Key staff from all participating agencies meet monthly to review project plans, goals and objectives.

PRELIMINARY RESULTS

Phase I. During the nine-month period between July 1, 1988 and March 31, 1989, 87 individuals were admitted into Phase I (Acton). Of this group 48% were white, 40% were Black, 10% were Hispanic and 2% were American Indian. The majority (82%) of the STHEP admittances to Acton were males. The modal age range was 25 to 34 years. Forty-nine percent completed Phase I and were transferred to the urban Mary Lind Alcohol Recovery Center (Phase

II), 23% are still in Phase I, and 28% did not complete Phase I. As of March 31, 1989, a total of 1,259 hours of group counseling, alcohol awareness and education, films, assertiveness training and relapse prevention, women's issues and AIDS education had been provided to STHEP residents during Phase I. STHEP residents also participated in 339 hours of individual counseling and had accumulated 3,802 contacts with AA meetings.

Phase II. During the six-month period between October 4, 1988 and March 31, 1989, 42 individuals were admitted into Phase II (Mary Lind) from Phase I (Acton). The majority (83%) were males. Sixty-six percent were Black, 24% white, 5% Hispanic and 5% American Indian. The modal age range was 32 to 38 years. Of the 42 individuals starting Phase II, 10 have completed, and 21 were still in the program as of April 1, 1989. Eleven participants (26%) did not complete Phase II. All 10 graduates were employed at time of program completion. Jobs held by these 10 individuals vary widely and include two plumbers, a landscaper, nursing home night supervisor, alcohol program advocate, cook, security guard, maintenance man and lab assistant.

Adjunct Support Services. During Phase I, all 87 individuals admitted into STHEP were screened for alcohol and drug abuse history, homeless background, legal history and current legal problems, educational backgrounds, and job skills. This information was gathered both formally in the initial intake interviews and on an on-going basis by the Project Coordinator and STHEP counselor during a participant's 90 day stay.

Participants who had not completed high school or who required up-grading of educational levels were referred to a basic skills education program conducted by Acton instructors. Medical and psychological evaluations were conducted for all STHEP participants as a prerequisite for State vocational rehabilitation assistance received during Phase II. Minor medical problems were handled at the on-site dispensary with referrals and transportation to the nearby Olive View Medical Center. Mental health needs were addressed through the provision of individual and/or group services by professional counselors at Acton, and additional mental health referrals were made as necessary to outside agencies.

IMPLEMENTATION ISSUES

During the first year of project implementation, three major barriers impacted project implementation: development of County contracts with sub-contractors, delay in State licensing of the Mary Lind facility, and replacement of the Evaluation Coordinator.

Development of Sub-Contracts

Upon receipt of the NIAAA grant on May 1, 1988, steps were immediately taken to develop a Memorandum of Understanding with the Acton program to provide Phase I of the project. Sub-contracts were also initiated with the Mary Lind Foundation, the Prevention Research Center and the California Association of Alcoholic Recovery Homes to provide other project services. The Memorandum was developed and finalized on July 1, 1988, when STHEP services at Acton were started. The sub-contracts with the other three agencies involved a lengthier and more complex process due to the specialized services offered by STHEP.

The Office of Alcohol Problems (OAP) has in place a specified contract format for its current set of services offered. The special relationships between contracting agencies, special services offered and data gathering components of STHEP were new to the OAP service system. New contract formats had to be developed, revised and approved by the Los Angeles County Counsel, Los Angeles Department of Health Services Contracts and Grants Office, the OAP community contract staff, the Alcohol and Drug Program Administration, Fiscal Administration Services staff, and finally, approved by the Board of Supervisors. The regular OAP contracting process for current services, from contract initiation to Board approval, takes about four to six weeks. The development of new contract services can take four to six months to complete. Efforts to develop the STHEP sub-contracts with the Mary Lind Foundation, the Prevention Research Center and the California Association of Alcoholic Recovery Homes were initiated in May of 1988, and completed at the end of September, 1988. Services for these components began in October, 1988.

Delay in State Licensing
of the Mary Lind Rena B. Facility

The Mary Lind Foundation began providing services to STHEP participants on October 4, 1988, five months after receipt of the grant award. The start-up timeline for the Mary Lind phase was three months after the Acton start-up to accommodate the first graduating group from the 90 day Acton STHEP program. The initial group of Acton graduates was transferred to the Mary Lind Foundation in October, 1988, with no actual delay in services. There was, however, a delay in the availability of the 99-bed Rena B. facility at the Mary Lind Foundation due to delays caused by State licensing requirements. The Rena B. facility was formally licensed and available for occupancy February 1, 1989. Until that time, Mary Lind STHEP participants were housed at an alternate site near the Rena B. facility.

Replacement of the Evaluation Coordinator

The sub-contract with the Pacific Institute for Research and Evaluation—Prevention Research Center was finalized on October 4, 1988. The Acton STHEP program had been providing services to STHEP participants since July 1, 1988. Thus, there was a three month lag in the implementation of evaluation activities. In the December report to NIAAA, the evaluation component continued to lag behind as a result of the delay in contract development. In addition, it became apparent that the geographical distance between the Northern California base of the evaluation coordinator and the Los Angeles project was a major obstacle to local evaluation staff training and supervision, data collection, and instrument development. In May, 1989, a local evaluator was hired to continue the implementation of the STHEP evaluation activities.

SUMMARY

The STHEP project is now fully operational and providing services to participants as planned. Participants are being served, system-linkages are being forged and evaluation of the process is ongoing.

REFERENCES

Kline, Michael V., Bacon, John D., Chinkin, Morris, and Manov, William F. (1987). "The client tracking system: A tool for studying the homeless," *Alcohol and Health Research World*, 11(3):66-68.

Lubran, Barbara G. (1987). "Alcohol-related problems among the Homeless: NIAAA's response," *Alcohol and Health Research World*, 11(3):4-8.

Wittman, Friedner D. (1989). Housing Models for Alcohol Programs Serving Homeless People, National Conference on Homelessness, Alcohol and Other Drugs, San Diego, CA February 2-4, 1989.

Louisville's Project Connect for the Homeless Alcohol and Drug Abuser

Gordon Scott Bonham, PhD
Diane E. Hague, MSSW
Millicent H. Abel, PhD
Patricia Cummings, MSSW
Richard S. Deutsch, PhD

Louisville is the largest city in Kentucky and is located on the Ohio River at the site of the only natural falls along the river. About two-thirds of a million people live in Louisville and the surrounding county, with a racial composition of approximately 84 percent white and 16 percent black. Louisville has few native Americans, Asians, or persons of Hispanic origin. The central business area of the city has experienced substantial business and cultural growth in recent years, but the transitional area around the central business district has decayed and is the home for most of the county's homeless. A number of missions, shelters, soup kitchens, and medical services are located in this area and are used by homeless people.

A Homeless Task Force was created in 1984 to coordinate services for the growing number of homeless people. The emphasis of the Task Force was on mental illness and homelessness, not on problems associated with homelessness and chemical abuse. Alcohol and drug treatment programs existed for indigent care, but were not specifically designed for the homeless. The alcohol and drug

Gordon Scott Bonham, Diane E. Hague, Patricia Cummings, and Richard S. Deutsch are affiliated with Seven Counties Services, Inc. and the University of Louisville. Millicent H. Abel is affiliated with the Urban Research Institute, University of Louisville, Louisville, KY 40292.

treatment programs which served the indigent were located in the downtown area in close proximity to shelters and food kitchens where the homeless congregate. However, the homeless chemically dependent were not staying in treatment long enough to help remedy their overall situation. In addition, the local shelters would not accept inebriated people. This left no place for the public inebriate except the jail, and jail overcrowding was becoming an important community concern. A sobering-up shelter was proposed by the city government in early 1987 as a way to solve jail overcrowding. The city proposed providing some case management services, but met with funding and zoning problems. Consequently, the shelter was not possible at that time. The Homeless Initiative of the National Institute on Alcohol Abuse and Alcoholism provided the opportunity to develop the services of Project Connect in response to these community needs and as a demonstration to determine if people who had basically "dropped out" could be helped to rejoin society.

Planning and program design for Project Connect began in late October 1987. At that time, both the Louisville Coalition for the Homeless and the Kentucky Division of Substance Abuse approached Seven Counties Services (SCS), the local community mental health agency, requesting that they submit a proposal for the NIAAA Homeless Initiative demonstration project funds.

Representatives from numerous agencies formed a planning group to review the existing services in the Louisville community for homeless alcohol and drug abusing individuals. These agencies included: Seven Counties Services, Louisville Coalition for the Homeless, Louisville City Government, Jefferson County Government, Salvation Army Adult Rehabilitation Center, St. John's Day Shelter, St. Vincent DePaul Society, Volunteers of America, Wayside Christian Mission, and the University of Louisville Urban Studies Center. The group developed a plan for providing and coordinating services which would fill the major service gaps in what the Louisville community was providing. Along with the program plan was an evaluation plan to provide data and information to help the community and nation address issues of planning, development, and provision of cost-effective services for the homeless with alcohol and drug problems.

The planning group identified the target population in Louisville, Kentucky, as homeless males with alcohol and/or drug problems. There was insufficient documentation of public inebriation among females to include them. Data collected from a mayor's task force on homelessness in 1985 identified approximately 2500 in this target group. The planning group decided to target homeless males cycling from shelters, food kitchens, and jails in order to intervene in that cycle and "connect" these individuals with other services. Thus, the name Project Connect was coined.

The planning group identified the following gaps in services that needed to be provided for the targeted population.

1. An entry point into services for men with alcohol problems who did not want formal detoxification treatment services.
2. An organized method of assisting homeless alcohol and drug dependent men to enter and use existing services, treatment programs, and self-help groups.
3. Work adjustment and vocational services which did not require residence in a specific domiciliary care or halfway house.
4. Formal linkages between identified "homeless" services and treatment services.
5. Information about what services alcohol and drug dependent homeless.
   men used and which services are effective and which are not.
6. Basic information about different subgroups of the alcohol and drug dependent homeless.

As a result of the planning group's recommendations, four agencies agreed to provide services proposed through Project Connect: Seven Counties (the community mental health and chemical dependency treatment agency) providing overall coordination for the project; Wayside Christian Mission, Inc., being responsible for a 24-hour Sobering-up Station and case management services; Volunteers of America providing work adjustment training and job placement; and the University of Louisville being responsible for research and evaluation of the program.

PROGRAM

Project Connect has three basic program components for the homeless man with alcohol and drug problems: a Sobering-up Station, case management, and work adjustment training. A liaison with the jail is considered a fourth component, although it links with the other three. The fifth component of Project Connect is agency linkage and coordination of services at the community level. The sixth component is the evaluation, a key task for a demonstration project.

Sobering-up Station

The Sobering-up Station is the entry point into Project Connect, and is the most publicly visible component. A four-room house, capable of sleeping 20, was specifically renovated for the Sobering-up Station. Completion of the renovation at the end of August 1988 inaugurated project services. The station is located on a side street, but in the same block as the other Wayside Christian Mission programs (Men's Night Shelter, Family Shelter). It is three blocks from the homeless day shelter and medical clinic, and six blocks from the hospital that serves the county's indigent population. The Project Connect station is the only shelter in the city that serves men when they are intoxicated.

During the first seven months of operation, the Sobering-up Station had 7309 admissions serving 669 different men. There was an average of 34 admissions per 24 hours of operation (18 admissions during the night and 16 during the day). The average length of stay was 10 to 12 hours. Since the beginning of the program, there has been a decrease in clients staying overnight and an increase in clients staying during the day hours only. Ninety percent of the men who utilized the Sobering-up Station came on their own, 4 percent were brought by the police, and the rest were referred by medical services, chemical dependency treatment services, and other shelters. Less than 2 percent of the admissions to the Sobering-up Station were men picked up by case managers in an outreach effort, and often these were specific men who were being targeted for services because of their frequent stays at the jail.

One-third (39%) of the men used the Sobering-up Station only once during the seven months of operation, and an additional one-fourth (25%) used it two to five times. There is a small group of men (11%) who used the station more than 25 times with an average of more than once a week. This group of frequent visitors is a major concern for project staff. Frequent use of the station can allow rapport and trust to develop with station workers and case managers, but could also be enabling these men to continue in their chemical abuse. The program staff is working on addressing this issue by developing procedures to limit visits to the station, and to begin motivating these individuals toward more responsibility for their own well-being.

Since opening, the Sobering-up Station has had to implement simple rules and policies to maintain order as well as to ensure the health and safety of both the men using the station and the staff. Basic rules require the men to shower and change clothes in order to control lice, and prohibit them from returning to the station within 24 hours after they leave.

The Sobering-up Station staff consist mostly of people recovering from their own alcohol and/or drug dependency. They have little formal education or chemical dependency training. They have been trained in basic shelter management, in handling disruptive behavior, and in basic first aid which includes cardio-pulmonary resuscitation (CPR). Police are called if disruptive behavior threatens to turn violent. Major medical emergencies are handled by calling Emergency Medical Services. Linkages between the police, the emergency room, and the project ensure smooth coordination.

Case Management

Case management is the core service of Project Connect. It is the service that "connects" the target population to other community resources. The men served by Project Connect have many needs and require consistent effort from case managers in assisting them toward a stable and productive life. The primary function of the case manager is to guide and encourage the clients to use services and resources available in the community, and to help the client connect into the already existing human services system. Project Connect's case management model is based on the principles that services should be tailored to meet the individual client's needs, they should focus on strengths rather than weaknesses, the case manager-client relationship is primary and essential, aggressive outreach is required, engaging clients in Alcoholics Anonymous and Narcotics Anonymous (AA/NA) is primary, and the community is an oasis of resources.

All clients are initially provided intensive case management services designed to give the men comprehensive support and encouragement to change their lives. An important part of the program is to recognize the men's abilities to change and to help build their self-esteem. It is an approach that requires aggressive outreach and small caseloads (20 per case manager) to be workable. Intensive case management is defined as client centered with the case manager ensuring that services are available rather than providing the services directly. Intensive case management requires almost daily contacts with clients but never less than twice a week. It requires staff review every three months, and active rather than reactive management. The approach involves extensive use of AA and NA with the case manager being aggressive in referring the men to meetings on a consistent basis and helping them obtain sponsors.

As the men become more stable, experience longer periods of sobriety, or live in halfway houses or other structured living programs, they are provided basic case management. This level of case management places greater responsibility on the individual to follow through on services, attend AA/NA, and maintain contact with the case manager. Men can move back and forth between intensive and basic case management according to their needs. Case management activities at both levels of intensity are shown in Table 1.

Project Connect originally proposed to provide assessment, service planning, and case management for 300 of the 900 men expected to be served at the Sobering-up Station. After seven months (March 1989), case managers were working with 67 clients. About three-fifths of these case management clients had entered case management by the end of the second month of the program. It soon became apparent that the original proposal of serving 300 men during two years was too ambitious to provide the intensity of case management services needed by the target population. While case management clients had the same age and racial distribution as the men being seen at the Station, both groups were older, experiencing

Table 1. Case Management Activities

---

o Admission: Interviewing, documenting initial needs,
                     completing paperwork

o Assessment: On-going process of evaluating chemical status,
                     health status, support systems, vocational
                     status, and environmental skills.

o Planning: Assisting clients to identify goals, specific
                     actions to reach and community services to use.

o Linking: Helping clients engage needed services by
                     identifying them, facilitating communication,
                     providing transportation, and coordinating
                     services.

o Monitoring: Ongoing assessment of clients' progress, needs,
                     and use of community resources.

o Tracking: Finding clients in their natural environment.

o Client Support   Enhancing clients' skills and understanding and
   and Education   developing trusting relationships.

o Case   Exchanging information with service providers to
   Consultation   assist in management of clients.

---

significantly more medical problems, and had longer histories of living on the street than originally projected. The target number was revised to 230 clients entering case management by the end of the second project year.

Recruitment into case management occurs in the Sobering-up

Station where case managers discuss needs and options with men eligible for case management. To be eligible for case management services the individual must:

1. Enter by way of the Sobering-up Station,
2. Be a male 18 years of age or older,
3. Be homeless (using the definition of homeless person from the Stewart B. McKinney Homeless Assistance Act P.L.100-77)
4. Have an alcohol or drug problem,
5. Not be transient, defined as living in the county for at least 45 days,
6. Not be experiencing a severe mental disorder that requires, or in the past has required, psychotropic drug treatment or inpatient psychiatric treatment.

Recruitment does not generally occur immediately. Some time is required to build a relationship with the client and develop his trust. Twenty-nine of the 67 men in case management were recruited on their first visit. However this was less than 4 percent of the men who had come to the Sobering-up Station during that time. Additional visits to the station increase the amount of contact the men have with the project and with case managers, and thereby increase the chances that they will agree to enter case management. A survival analysis technique projects that one-fourth of the men will agree to case management by the time they have come to the Station 30 times.

A problem was recognized fairly early in the program – an increasing proportion of the visits to the Sobering-up Station were being made by men who had already agreed to case management. A decision was made to limit the number of clients in case management and to change its intensity. Case managers would spend less time talking to men who were not in case management and more time working with those who had already agreed to the program.

Use of the Sobering-up Station by case management clients has not changed much, but, there are indications that case management clients are making progress. According to the case managers' monthly evaluations of the clients, only one client in ten (10%) who was in case management during October had spent every night off the street in some type of appropriate shelter. (See Table 2.) By February, half (49%) of the clients had spent every night off the street. Weather may have had some influence on this change, but a mild winter leaves open the possibility that the program was having an increasing affect on the men's living situation. A second key indicator of progress is the percent of men who were judged by the case managers to have been "clean and dry" (without chemical use) during the whole month. Only one client in 12 (8%) was judged to have been clean and dry in October, while one in four (24%) was judged to have been clean and dry during March. The other columns in the table, while also indicators of client outcomes, may more appropriately indicate changes in case managers' expectations. One-fourth (23%) of the clients in October were viewed by the case managers as complying with their service plans, even though a much smaller percent were off the street the whole month, or were off alcohol and chemicals the whole month. In March, case managers felt only one in 12 clients (8%) was making excellent progress, even though two in five were off the street and one-fourth

Table 2. Percent of Case Management Clients by

Monthly Outcome Indicators

Month	# Days On Street	Clean and Dry	Admits Problem	Comply with Plan	Making Excellent Progress	# of Client Reports
Oct(88)	10	8	28	23	15	(39)
Nov	19	16	28	16	16	(57)
Dec	27	18	18	13	16	(62)
Jan(89)	35	17	24	13	14	(63)
Feb	49	22	19	8	10	(63)
March	42	24	20	12	8	(66)

were clean and dry the whole month. A number of things had happened about the first of January: the intensity of case management increased, recruitment of new cases was restricted, 15 (22%) of the case management clients were accepted as lost, and it was recognized the rest had been in case management for several months. All these factors appear to have increased case managers' expectations of the clients more rapidly than the clients were changing, lowering case manager evaluations of client progress.

One objective in case management is to implement service plans that connect the men to appropriate community services including inpatient detoxification and rehabilitation, aftercare, out-patient counseling, domiciliary care, transitional living care, and other social service and health care. During the period of January through March 1989, 617 agency contacts were recorded on behalf of the 67 clients in case management. All clients in case management had service plans developed. Through the first seven months of the program, 480 service plan activities or referrals had been developed, an average of seven per case management client. The largest category of activities or referrals (156) were for medical and health services, with over half of these for chemical dependency treatment. The remaining service plan activities or referrals were about evenly divided among the remaining three categories of employment/economic, housing/shelter, and support systems.

Three full-time case managers and one part-time case manager were hired during the first months of the Project Connect and began working as case managers when the Sobering-up Station was opened. The characteristics, training, and retention of case managers became a major issue for the project during the subsequent nine months. One of the case managers resigned in October 1988 due to health problems and two resigned in April and May 1989 to take other positions. It is now recognized that as new case managers take their places, they need to be trained to deal realistically with the slow progress of the client population and to understand that the manager's role is to connect the men to services, not to provide the services. All of the original case managers were men, and three were recovering alcoholics. Project management now feels there needs to be a balance among case management staff as to gender, recovering status, and personality (i.e., nurturers and confronters).

Jail Liaison

Part of Project Connect includes a liaison between the jail, the case managers, and the Sobering-up Station. A jail liaison was hired in the sixth month of the project after a formal linkage agreement was finalized between Project Connect and jail officials. The jail liaison meets individually with each homeless incarcerated male with alcohol or related charges, explains the services available through Project Connect, and refers him to the Sobering-up Station. The jail liaison works with the case managers to track case management clients who return to jail, and with advocates of the court system to have the men referred back to the project. The jail liaison also identifies men who are jailed frequently in order to target these men for case management services. The jail liaison started in November, and during the first seven months of his work, he had 527 contacts with 121 homeless men in the jail who were mainly charged with alcohol intoxication.

An agreement has recently been reached with the judicial system to allow court-ordered case management from Project Connect for individuals who are chronic public inebriates and who consistently use the jail as a way station. If one of these individuals comes before the court, the jail liaison will ask the prosecuting attorney and the judge to formally order case management. If the man fails to comply, he will be given time to serve. The liaison has the responsibility to notify the court of noncompliance. The agreement stipulates that the court will then issue and enforce a bench warrant for the individual's arrest. The use of coercive intervention appears to be a necessary part of working with some of the most chronic public inebriates.

Vocational Training Program

Vocational training and job placement is a major goal of the program for men who can maintain sobriety for a period of time. Many of the case management clients, however, are not candidates for employment because of age, physical or medical conditions, or cognitive abilities, and therefore are not placed in the vocational program. Men receiving case management services are briefly interviewed by the Volunteers of America staff at the Sobering-up

Station site as soon as possible to determine whether or not they are candidates for employment and what will be necessary before they are ready for vocational training. These brief interviews with 56 men found 16 to be potential candidates for vocational training services once they achieved a 90-day sobriety requirement.

After six months of operation, the vocational component has provided job training for seven men. Four of the seven men completed the training and were placed in jobs, and all four successfully achieved their 30-day job retention. The job training staff of the vocational program closely monitors each man's progress and gives him the close attention he needs to succeed in the program. The vocational program also provides small financial incentives for men while attending the classes and a $50 bonus for retaining the job for 30 days. Some of the men, however, have been unhappy about the length of time between starting the program and obtaining a job.

Originally, 120 of the 300 expected case management clients were to be referred to work adjustment training, with 80 projected to actually complete the training. It is now projected that 30 men will complete the program during the first two years and achieve long-term employment. A major problem with the vocational program goals was the mistaken assumption that public inebriate men could meet the requirements for entering the vocational program in the first year. Experience suggests that the vocational component should not have begun until the second year of the project. Additionally, a number of training and vocational options may need to be available to interest the men.

ORGANIZATION AND COMMUNITY OWNERSHIP

The organization, coordination, and community ownership of Project Connect operate at several levels. These levels are all required to secure the success of the project. The executive directors and the Project Connect managers from each of the four agencies (Wayside Christian Mission, Seven Counties Services, Volunteers of America, and the Urban Studies Center at the University of Louisville) meet monthly to review the progress of the program, discuss problems, and plan for the coming month. This meeting is chaired by the principal investigator, the director of the Seven Counties Services' Alcohol and Drug Program. The chief evaluator normally has data to share at this meeting and deals as well with any problems in the research/evaluation area.

The project director, who reports directly to the principal investigator, meets with the project managers of the Sobering-up Station and case management component, the vocational training component, and the evaluation component once a month. The jail liaison, who is directly supervised by the project director, also attends these meetings. These meetings focus entirely on issues in day-to-day operations. These meetings ensure that communication channels remain open between the different components; and if problems arise, they can quickly be resolved.

Client case review meetings are held weekly by the project director, who has experience in chemical treatment programs, with the case managers, the Sobering-up Station/case management supervisor, the vocational counselor, and the evaluation data coordinator. The progress of selected case management clients is discussed in these meetings. The case managers and shelter workers have their own weekly meetings to coordinate services and discuss specific problems which may exist in the Sobering-up Station.

Project Connect has an Advisory Council, formed in August 1988, which meets once a month. The 22-member Council consists of the four directors of the agencies directly involved in Project Connect, five representatives from the criminal justice system (judge, jail staff, police captain, crime commission, district attorney's office), representatives from five other agencies who provide services to the homeless, the assistant director of the local housing authority, head nurse from the hospital emergency room serving the indigent, two representatives from the local government, two representatives from other parts of the University of Louisville (Medical School and School of Social Work), a representative from the City Business Association, and the chair of the neighborhood association where the Sobering-up Station is located. The purpose of the Council is to foster broad community ownership, coordination, and input to Project Connect. The Council members have given input on avoiding potential problem areas and enhancing the visibility of the project.

The formation of the Advisory Council is one way of fostering community participation. The members of the Council represent a broad cross-section of the community. The goal is for every agency or group represented to feel partnership in the project. In addition, there has been extensive publicity about the project that has been geared to general citizen awareness and ownership. Since the start of the project there have been five articles in the local newspaper, six stories on the local evening news and one story on a local morning news program. Local government officials participated in the open house for the Sobering-up Station. Project staff have also made special efforts to ensure that U.S. Congressmen and Senators from the area are kept well informed of Project Connect activities and status.

EVALUATION

The evaluation for Project Connect includes both process evaluation and outcome evaluation (process and outcome variables), relates to two classes of actors (clients and agencies), and uses two types of methods (quantitative and qualitative). Client outcomes relate to their achievement of program goals and to changes in their quality of life. Agency outcomes relate to agency interaction and to agency staff attitudes and behavior toward clients and other human service workers. Each set of outcomes (client and agency) is expected to be influenced by processes associated with the program components implemented as part of Project Connect. The multiple method approach of using both quantitative and qualitative methods to measure processes and outcomes provides exact measurement and vivid description. Quantitative methods include face-to-face pre- and post-interview data with clients, monthly program data on clients, self-administered pre- and post-questionnaire data for community agency staff, and selected administrative record data from Project Connect agencies. Qualitative methods include ethnographic observation and interviews and journals maintained by immediate program personnel. Data collection instruments were designed cooperatively by the program and evaluation staff so they could meet the needs of both.

Quantitative Measurement

Client Data Collection

Alcohol and drug abusing men are initially exposed to Project Connect through the Sobering-up Station. Data are collected on these individuals through a Shelter Intake Log. These client data are used for programmatic purposes (e.g., client screening for the case management program) and for evaluation purposes (e.g., monitoring of Sobering-up Station utilization). Men are assigned identification numbers upon entering the Sobering-up Station for the first time, and this identification is used to track individuals and the services they receive throughout all components of Project Connect.

When a man agrees to case management, he is interviewed by the case manager using the Addiction Severity Index (ASI) (McLellan, Luborsky, O'Brien & Woody, 1980) and by an evaluation team member using a client interview questionnaire. Case management clients will be followed a maximum of 19 months, depending upon when they entered the program. Monthly Client Evaluations, which provide immediate outcome data, are completed for each client by their case managers. At the end of the project, a second wave of interviews will be conducted by evaluation team members with all clients who entered case management regardless of whether they are still active in the program. Those clients selected for the vocational training program (i.e., those who qualify on a work program screening form) complete short questionnaires before and after the training. Clients are evaluated weekly throughout the vocational training with a client progress evaluation form. When the client is placed in a job, the employer completes a job placement confirmation form. After four weeks on the job, the employer completes a 30-day retention form and assesses the client's behavior on the job through a progress evaluation form. Secondary data will also be collected on the case management clients. These data include (a) number of jail visits to the clients by the jail liaison, (b) jail history for the years prior to and during Project Connect, and (c) medical history, obtained from medical and emergency room records in cooperation with the Homeless Health Care Program.

Agency Data Collection

Staff of service providers who work with homeless alcoholic and drug abusing men were asked to complete a self-administered questionnaire prior to the implementation of Project Connect. A second survey will be conducted 12 months later. The primary purpose of the survey is to determine how staffs of these agencies are affected by Project Connect. Participants included paid and volunteer, fulltime and part-time staff, from (a) government service providers and parent agencies, (b) public safety agencies, (c) short-term direct service agencies, (d) medical and emergency agencies, and (e) counseling and behavior modification agencies. Preliminary analyses of the before-program questionnaire data reveal a generally negative perception of homeless men with alcohol and drug problems by these staffs and suggest that organized interaction and cooperation among the agencies are minimal. Comparisons at pre- and postprogram responses will determine whether the staff views of homeless alcoholic and drug abusing men change, and whether agency networking activities increase, decrease, or stay the same during the year following the introduction of Project Connect.

Agency level data are also being collected on the case managers' use of their time. The case managers' actual time spent in several categories of services and for each client are recorded on individual daily activities logs. The categories of services on the log were coordinated with three other demonstration projects, although they are not identical. This coordination will allow some cross-program comparisons of case management.

Client Outcomes Measures

The primary client outcomes for Project Connect are derived from changes between the initial interview and the second interview relative to the items presented below:

• extent of alcohol and drug use
• quality of life, e.g., general well-being, self-care behavior
• physical health and mental health status, e.g., extent of doctor's care; diagnostic and perceived health, demoralization, hopelessness
• economic status, e.g., efforts in obtaining employment and/or entitlements
• arrests
• access to shelter, housing, health, and counseling/treatment services, e.g., number of services used; self-rating of access after program

Client-Related Process Measures

Two types of client process measures are included in the study: internal program processes which document the dynamics of involvement with the Sobering-up Station, case management, and vocational training program, and external processes which may contaminate or accentuate program processes. Process items included in Project Connect include:

• number of times client uses the Sobering-up Station
• perceived quality of care in the Sobering-up Station
• length of time in case management and amount of contact between case manager and client
• characteristics of service plan and extent to which client follows treatment plan
• extent and type of alcohol and drug services utilized
• amount of contact case manager has with service providers
• perceived quality of case management and services provided by community agencies
• number of changes in housing arrangements
• participation in the vocational training program
• skill level changes resulting from the vocational training
• number of stressful events on the street, e.g., incidents of victimization and illness, weather, and jailings
• relationship with friends

Agency Process Measures

Agency process measures involve:

- number of referrals of program clients to agencies
- number of general contacts or exchanges by the program with agencies

Agency Outcomes Measures

Agency outcome measures relate to two goals for improving service delivery through Project Connect, and include:

- agency staffs' perceptions of and behavior toward the homeless who have alcohol- and drug-related problems
- levels of cooperation and formal linkages and networking among staff of agencies that provide services

Qualitative Component

Ethnographic research provides a firsthand description of life on the streets for homeless men. Their perception of life, the community, and services available to them will be described, analyzed, and integrated with quantitative measures. Ethnography's traditional strength is its ability to analyze and represent the perceptions of different groups involved in the same social setting. Evaluation of Project Connect, which involves complex interpersonal and organizational interaction and multiple influences on individual clients, calls for the use of ethnographic methods of observation and informal interviewing as part of an integrated evaluation plan. The ethnographic component is designed to maximize the evaluator's access to data not obtainable through quantitative methods alone.

The first phase of the ethnographic research involved general observation of street life and informal interviews with homeless men on the perceptions they had of themselves and others. These activities occurred prior to the visible start of Project Connect. Some of the informants may never participate in Project Connect, but their information complements the evaluation of the project as a measure of why some men choose not to participate. The second phase of the ethnographic research examines case management clients. Both observation and informal interviews are being used to gain insight into the client's perception of the program and how it does (or does not) work. A number of men will be followed throughout the project, but tracking these men is extremely time consuming as they do not stay in the same place. Sufficient time is essential in ethnographic research; the details of a person's life may not be obtained in one week, one month, or perhaps even in nine months. The third phase of the ethnographic research involves the interactions and perceptions of the Sobering-up Station staff and case managers with the clients which are being examined through observation and a structured interview.

Another aspect of the qualitative evaluation involves describing the implementation of Project Connect and analyzing how the implementation followed or differed from the original design. Information for this analysis will come from monthly reports prepared by each component manager and the journals kept by key program and evaluation personnel. The almost daily contact between program and evaluation staff is an important mechanism for communicating program processes. Joint involvement in analysis and evaluation issues ensures that important details are not overlooked.

CONCLUSION

There is a popular image in America that homeless men are "bums" and "derelicts" who have fallen to the bottom of life out of laziness and self-pity. Working people see them loitering drunkenly on the street, or sitting and staring, and perhaps, on occasion, fighting or causing some other disturbance. Community residents may become concerned only when approached for money on the street, or when some form of other social problem is attributed to "bums" or "derelicts." For human service providers, however, the homeless alcoholic and drug abusers present a complex set of problems that remain largely unsolved by traditional service delivery. Generally the homeless have none of the residential, family, work, or institutional links to the community on which most human service agencies rely. The question for both the human service agencies and for society at large, is what can be done for these people and what is feasible?

Project Connect is a federally funded demonstration project to determine if case management services, supported by a sobering-up shelter as an entry point and a vocational program as the exit point, can help homeless alcoholic and drug abusing men in Louisville to become productive members of the larger community. The project was designed to utilize the experiences and expertise of four community agencies in addressing the problems of intervening with homeless chemical-abusing men. The project services, however, are only supplemental because the program was designed to connect the men to the existing community services and resources that they needed. The involvement of multiple agencies with different perspectives in the project presents special problems as well as special opportunities. Communication is very important, and a balance must be maintained among different value systems and approaches to problems. Balance also must be maintained between program provision and evaluation if knowledge is to be expanded.

Will Project Connect work? It is too soon to tell. Homeless alcoholic and drug abusing men have their own set of values and perceptions about what life holds for them. To understand them, to work with them, or to change them requires time and intimate knowledge of their lives. Some early expressions obtained through the ethnographic evaluation component suggest that the project can expect to fail in its stated objectives, to be ignored as irrelevant, and to be successful, all at the same time. Before the Sobering-up Station opened, the publicly inebriated man either slept in an alley or old building, or, if unlucky enough to get caught (or lucky, depending on one's point of view), would spend the night in jail (fondly referred to as the "Cross Bar Hotel"). The Station was immediately seen by the homeless alcoholic as a place to go to avoid problems with the police, the mission, or the troublemakers on the street. To the drunks, the rules at this Sobering-up Station were not strict. Indeed, the Station lacked the formal bureaucratic rules of other missions or institutions. If you got drunk, you walked in, gave your name and birth date (if capable) and either went to bed or ate and cleaned up a bit then slept it off. When you awoke, you could sit around the Station or simply leave. One man described what it enabled him to do:

This is great! If I get loaded now I can sleep it off in there and not worry about getting rolled (robbed). Of course, I'm usually too wasted to worry about that shit anyway. But it's good they've opened a drunk tank up. Why'd they do it? I guess they figured too many winos were trying to sneak into the mission. God save 'em!

As with most new programs, Project Connect evolved as it was implemented. Rules by the Station workers eventually emerged that affected the attitudes street men had toward the Station. Rules are necessary in any organization to keep some order and some hierarchy of authority. The Sobering-up Station developed simple rules to keep men under control and assert authority (and also to eliminate lice). After a month of operation, shelter workers required men to shower and change clothes when entering (if they were not too drunk) and then sleep for an hour or more before receiving any food. Rowdiness was cause for expulsion. The loosely organized drunk tank was tightening up and, in the eyes of some homeless men, becoming one more agency to deal with. As one man lamented:

It's become another piece of bureaucratic crap. They want me to be interviewed, for what? I know who I am and what I do. And I know about statistics, I have a degree in business from . . . They'll set up these interviews, make me a number and what do I get? A waste of time, and Bob here feels the same.

These views, that the program enables the continuation of the problem or is a waste of time, are not held by all men. The ones who became participants in the case management component and made an effort, believe it is a saving grace. One such man had been seen sober only once during the ethnographer's first nine months on the street. The man's early thoughts on the program were:

Those people don't know how to help. Why would they want to help me? Who the hell pays them to do that? I don't believe they could do anything for me. Right now the best damn thing they could do would be to give me a fuckin' drink. Damn, I need it. And I hear they will take the bottle from you. Is that help? God no!

Later he signed up for case management. At first, during withdrawal, he was very angry. But after three weeks' sobriety, he openly discussed how he was feeling:

I knew they had something here but I just never did anything. My whole life has been drinking, nothing but. I just started thinking that it's really killing me. Look at me now, I'm turning yellow and I can feel my liver hurtin'! I hope I can stay off of it and find a job. I used to work on Harley's, but I think the wine has killed my brain that I can't remember what to do.

This man is one who is meeting with some success for now. Only time will tell how long his success will last or if he ever will recover. Only time will tell whether he is unique, or if there will be many more like him.

REFERENCES

McLellan, A. T., L. Luborsky, C. P. O'Brien, and G. E. Woody. (1980) An improved evaluation instrument for substance abuse patients: The Addiction Severity Index. *Journal of Nervous and Mental Disorders*, 168, 26-33.

Community Treatment
of the Chronic Public Inebriate I:
Implementation

Mark L. Willenbring, MD
Joseph A. Whelan, MSSA
James S. Dahlquist, JD
Michael E. O'Neal, MA

The term chronic public inebriate (CPI) refers to that combination of chronic alcohol abuse, unemployment, homelessness, poverty, and poor physical and emotional health that has proved to be one of society's most vexing problems. Also known as skid-row, or chronic recidivist alcoholics, individuals leading this life are often highly visible through their public behavior and extensive use of public services. In Hennepin County (Minneapolis), approximately 850 people could be considered CPIs at any one time, using the arbitrary cutting point of 15 + lifetime admissions to the Alcohol Receiving Center (detoxification center). Approximately 450 of these individuals are "active" (drinking and presenting themselves to social services) at any one time (Minnesota Institute of Public Health, 1986). American Indians are grossly overrepresented among CPI's in Hennepin County, even though Indians comprise 43% of the CPI's in Hennepin County, which is 66 times higher than would be expected based on their representation in the general population (Minnesota Institute of Public Health, 1986). The CPI

Mark L. Willenbring is affiliated with the Chemical Health Division, Hennepin County, Minnesota, and the Department of Psychiatry, University of Minnesota, Minneapolis, MN. Joseph A. Whelan, James S. Dahlquist, and Michael E. O'Neal are affiliated with the Chemical Health Division, Hennepin County, MN. Lisa Miller assisted with data entry and analysis.

utilizes public services significantly out of proportion to his numbers, and accounts for a disproportionate share of alcoholism treatment costs (Wells, 1985). CPIs have excess medical morbidity (Ashley et al., 1976), resulting in high medical (Weiller, 1978; McIntosh, 1982) and psychiatric (Woogh, 1986; Miller et al., 1984; Schwartzburg and Schwartz, 1976) service utilization, and excess morbidity (Combs-Orme et al., 1983). In the feasibility study for this project completed in 1984 (Minnesota Institute of Public Health, 1986), we determined the service utilization patterns and associated costs over a one year period in 1984-5 for 43 CPI's randomly selected from the detox center population. Detox, medical, and psychiatric costs totalled $15,900 per person per year, and expenditures for legal and social services amounted to $6,940 per person per year, for total expenditures of $22,840, per person per year. Thus, total public expenditures that we could directly account for amounted to over $9.7 million per year for less than 500 people in one urban county alone.

Unfortunately, it is now clear that, although many types of treatments have been attempted, and some approaches have shown promise in some areas, there are no comprehensive treatments for the CPI with demonstrated effectiveness (Richman and Neumann, 1984; Finn, 1985; Annis and Smart, 1976; Ditman et al., 1967). The experience in Hennepin County is illustrative.

The Chronic Options Team was formed in 1985 to provide a more coordinated response to the chronic public inebriate. The goals of the Team were to (1) intervene forcefully in the public drinking pattern of the chronic public inebriate, (2) use a clinical team of substance abuse counselors and service providers to assess client needs and plan treatment, (3) offer a range of recovery services, (4) coordinate treatment and movement of clients through the service network, and (5) develop cooperative agreements among caregivers to ensure client acceptance and payment for service.

In 1986, the Chronic Options Team made 636 referrals to five residential facilities. At any point in time, approximately 275 clients were in residential care. The team approach allowed a County staff of 4 to manage, on an episodic basis, the 850 clients defined as chronic public inebriates. Systematic analysis of the County's experience, however, indicated that the episodic intervention strategy was not having the desired impact on the most frequent users of the detoxification facility (a subgroup of 450 chronic recidivist alcoholics) and that continued expenditures were not warranted. The revolving door of the drunk tank had been replaced by more costly revolving doors at detox centers and other treatment facilities. This experience and the continuing need to respond to the problem of chronic alcoholism, suggests that more effective treatment models must be developed.

Three fundamental errors appear to have contributed to past failures with this population. First, the fact that the CPI is severely and chronically disabled in multiple areas of life (Bahr, 1969; Blumberg et al., 1971; Roth and Bean, 1985; Bassuk et al., 1984; Cohen and Sokolovsky, 1983; Myerson and Mayer, 1966; Ashley et al., 1971; Blower, 1978; Neuner and Schultz, 1986) has often not been fully appreciated. Planners and caregivers have tended to place too great an emphasis on alcoholism, with the underlying assumption that if the alcohol were removed, the other problems would go away (Finn, 1985).

Second, this approach has led to setting unrealistically high goals. Most programs have attempted to fully rehabilitate the CPI, to the point of long-term, independent living (Finn, 1985; Kurtz and Reiger, 1975; Annis and Smart, 1976; Ditman et al., 1967), after only a few weeks or months of treatment. It is our contention that the CPI has himself demonstrated that that goal is unrealistic. It would appear that treatment goals appropriate for a chronic illness (i.e., modifying the course, alleviating suffering) are more applicable.

Finally, based on the above assumptions, treatment models that have been used for the CPI have been those found most useful in the middle-class, non-alienated alcoholic. Programs often last only a few weeks or months, and typically involve a period of residential care. Many programs appear unable or unwilling to change programs to fit the client. Almost all assume or require motivation on the part of the client, and many discontinue treatment if the client relapses. This analysis suggests that in order for treatment to be successful, it would have to be (1) based upon a realistic assessment of the characteristics and needs of the CPI; (2) not biased by a particular treatment philosophy, but rather flexibly responsive to the population needs; (3) realistic in goals and expectations regarding program outcome; (4) long term in focus; and (5) comprehensive in scope.

Intensive case management (ICM) is a community based treatment which has been shown to be effective with people with chronic mental illness (Stein and Test, 1984). Individuals with chronic mental illness resemble CPIs in that (1) they also suffer from a severe, chronic stigmatizing disorder, characterized by remissions and relapses, for which no curative treatment is available, which then produces (2) chronic disability in multiple life areas, and (3) chronic dependence on social welfare institutions. These similarities suggest that ICM may be a useful tool in the long-term supportive treatment of the homeless CPI. This paper describes the development and early implementation of a demonstration project which utilizes an ICM system for the CPI based on these principles.

MODEL DESCRIPTION

We have adapted a model of ICM that was developed in Madison, Wisconsin, by Stein and Test (Stein and Test, 1980; Weisbrod et al., 1980). Central to this model is the core services team (Test, 1979) that performs assessment, planning, resource development, implementation, and review functions. This team carries the responsibility of making sure that the client's needs are met. The target of services is thus the whole client. This does not mean that the team will provide all of the services, but rather that they can never transfer this responsibility to someone else. This results in a team that is function-specific, rather than facility-specific, and provides continuity of care. That is, they stick with the client whether the client improves or deteriorates, so the client has a consistent resource.

There are several ways to structure case management, varying from individual primary case management to programs where responsibility for each client is diffused throughout the team (Reinke and Greenley, 1986). We elected to use the modified team approach, where there is a primary case manager who can form a long-term relationship with the client, but the team also takes significant responsibility, in order to avoid overwhelming individual case managers. This is a very active, street-oriented form of case management, where the case managers are out looking for their clients when they do not know where they are. The small caseload makes it possible to devote considerable time and energy to each active client. Case managers advocate for clients' needs, and assist clients to obtain needed services. They monitor the response to a referral or intervention, and intervene again if need be. Even when a client is referred to a facility or program, the case manager does not stop being involved. Frequent face-to-face visits are usual.

A tier system has been developed to serve as an outline for classifying client problem severity. The severity of the drinking problem and social stability are both rated, and combined to classify the client into a tier. The tier level then is used to suggest the level and types of interventions appropriate. Once validated, this may serve as a useful guide to others who may wish to replicate this model, in whole or in part. We are currently working to refine this system, which is described in the "Borrow Me a Quarter" feasibility study (Neuner and Schultz, 1986).

The characteristics of ICM outlined above include several elements previously shown useful in treating CPIs. In particular, a common denominator in most treatment programs exhibiting some success has been the establishment of an enduring caring relationship with the CPI (Bates, 1983; Moos et al., 1978). Establishing this relationship must often involve "enforced contact," with significant activity on the part of the provider; simply offering the opportunity to relate to someone has not proved useful (Pittman, 1974; Annis and Smart, 1976; Ogbourne and Collier, 1979). Services need to address broad social welfare needs, especially housing, as well as drinking behavior (Finn, 1985; Blower, 1978; Zimberg, 1974). It may be helpful to make resource availability contingent upon behavior change (Miller, 1975), so we have begun focusing on money management as a potential tool. While use of coercion has been shown to be helpful by several investigators (Lovald and Stub, 1968; Baker, 1985; Rosenberg and Liftik, 1976; Pratt, 1976), we have not found coercion particularly useful. We will, however, periodically hold someone for brief periods (a few days), in order to prevent severe physical and psychiatric deterioration. For those CPI's who are in a period of remission, or who perhaps identify with more dominant values, programs providing a community (e.g., Salvation Army) have proved somewhat effective (Moos et al., 1978).

The potential advantages of this type of program for the CPI are as follows: It should reduce fragmentation of care, and create an incentive among case managers to find or create innovative solutions to problems, because they cannot "dump" the client on another agency. It should promote comprehensive assessment and planning, a proactive, assertive therapeutic approach, and a long-term, realistic view of what will be needed to support this client in the community. Rather than preparing the client for living in the community, the focus is on maintaining the client in the community.

Local Development of the Model

The Community Treatment of the Chronic Public Inebriate Model was developed over a six year period. Conceptual development began as a series of conversations between the senior author and Dr. Leonard I. Stein about adapting the Training in Community Living Model for Chronic Public Inebriates. Dr. Stein helped develop and ran the Training in Community Living project, considered one of the most successful community treatment programs for the chronically mentally ill (Langsely, 1985; Stein and Test, 1980; Weisbrod et al., 1980; Test, 1979). Conceptual development continued under the auspices of the Minneapolis Advisory Committee on Drug and Alcohol Problems. A feasibility study funded by the Minnesota Division of Chemical Dependency, the Minneapolis Community Development Agency, the Minneapolis Police Department, and the Minneapolis Foundation, took place from April-December, 1985. Officials of Hennepin County, who operate the ARC and other treatments for CPIs, as well as the Minnesota Division of Chemical Dependency, were heavily involved in the subsequent planning, execution, and interpretation of the study. The study's conclusion was that intensive case management showed excellent feasibility for the CPI, and should be tried.

A grant from the Minnesota Division of Chemical Dependency for funding for a pilot project was funded at the level of $30,000 in

November, 1987, to begin in January, 1988. The funding was to enable the Hennepin County Chemical Health Division to hire two case managers, and to send them to Madison, Wisconsin, for training in the community treatment model, along with one supervisor. Due to a variety of administrative problems, this grant was only partially implemented, and never fully funded. However, it did allow us to assess early hiring and training methods. Finally, funds for this demonstration project became available through the Stuart B. McKinney Homeless Assistance Act.

The primary goals of this project are to develop an innovative treatment to homeless chronic public inebriates, to document and evaluate its effectiveness, and to do so in a way so as to facilitate replication elsewhere. Other goals include coordination and stimulation of resources for our clients, especially housing, and health and mental health services. Improving the functioning of the client is the ultimate goal for the clinical program; this will, in turn, lead to improved quality of life and economic well being. We will also assess the implementation, relative efficacy and efficiency of ICM, as compared to non-intensive case management (NICM), and also to the current approaches being utilized to treat the CPI in Hennepin County (Episodic Care; EC).

IMPLEMENTATION

Hiring and Training Staff

Two case managers were hired under the pilot project funded by the Minnesota Division of Chemical Dependence and undertook the training in the ICM model in Madison, Wisconsin. Before the case managers began taking clients, problems developed in the funding for the project, and the project was never fully funded. Not having the pilot project in place has meant that we have had to implement this project without the benefit of having the pilot in place for several months beforehand. This resulted in some minor delays in implementation, compared to projections. The current Project Director began work in August after a previously selected candidate declined the position in June. The Research Coordinator started at the same time. The remainder of the case management team was hired in August and started in September. Overall, the project lost about a month in the implementation of the program.

Orientation to the project and to Hennepin County's structure, rules, and services took place during the first week of employment. The staff spent the second week in Madison learning about the ICM model. The training that took place was a hybrid training developed with Dane County Mental Health Center and a detoxification center program in Madison that utilized some case management. The training appeared to be successful in meeting its goals of team formation and inculcation of case management principles.

Training of case managers has continued primarily through inservice education and clinical supervision. The senior author initially met with the case management staff weekly to discuss implementation of the model. More recently, the Project Director and a Unit Supervisor have had the primary responsibility of translating the concept into action through clinical supervision of line staff. Staff turnover has been an issue. Three of the original five case managers left the Project between December and February. The resignations occurred for a variety of reasons but had the singular effect of further delaying project implementation.

The current group of case managers consists of three entry-level chemical health counselors, one bachelor-level social worker, and one case manager hired as a bachelor-level social worker, but who has a background as a chemical health counselor. Three are women, and one (male) is of Native American descent. All others are White. The unit supervisor is a White male with a master's-level counselling degree, with a background in chemical health and experience with CPIs in Madison (thus, he is also familiar with the the ICM model). The team appears to be functioning well.

Community Outreach and Linkage

Community outreach began within the Minnesota Division of Chemical Dependence with the hiring of the first case managers for the non-intensive case management group in May 1988. Some existing Alcohol Receiving Center (ARC) staff resisted the implementation of this program. Resistance seemed to be on both conceptual and personal bases. This resistance culminated in February, 1989, when some ARC staff issued a "report" which was critical of the new project and concluded that current county treatment approaches were better. In response, the Director of the Minnesota Division of Chemical Dependence and the ARC Program Manager reiterated their support for the demonstration project, and made it clear that this kind of resistance would not be allowed to continue. This point appeared to be a watershed, and, in conjunction with other events of the time, marked the end of early implementation. In many ways, the first task of any new program within an existing division is to survive, to find a place and be accepted within the existing structure. Failure to accomplish this leads to crisis management, and hampers the ability to stabilize program operations. At the time this occurred, logs from the PI, Evaluation Director and Program Director all indicate a decision to avoid being distracted by ARC staff actions, and to concentrate instead on implementing program goals.

While these and other basic implementation issues took precedence during the first few months, community outreach has also occurred outside the Division, beginning especially around November 1988. The Citizens' Advisory Council was established in December 1988, and has met 3 times. Other efforts have focused initially on the criminal justice system and housing. These efforts have involved (1) clarifying the way each system works, and how it affects the program's clients, (2) educating the systems about the clientele, and (3) advocating for changes in the system of care that would benefit our clients. The efforts appear to be having some effect, although it is too early to see more than modest results.

Clinical Operations

The ICM team began taking cases in the last week of September. Over the next two months, 56 clients were recruited. During this time, the case management team developed and refined intake procedures and initial treatment planning and interventions. Treatment plans were developed on all clients within a month of first contact, and are being reevaluated every 6 months. This part of the operation appears to be functioning smoothly. Case managers report feeling comfortable with the procedures that are in place. Examination of the time reporting by case managers indicates that there has been a progression of clinical time spent on screening/evaluation from 25% initially, to 46%, and then to around 10% at the current time.

Intake of clients was stopped after December, when the caseload was 56 (or 11/cases mgr). This was done in order to give case managers time to begin treating and stabilizing a severely disordered group of clients. Team turnover contributed to the need for this. The team is now planning on beginning recruitment again within the next few weeks, in order to bring the caseload up to the optimal level (which is expected to be about 15).

One complication that arose had to do with a potential selection bias in the comparison among case management groups. Changes in protocol necessitated by the early introduction of one of the control groups might lead to selection bias by post-randomization screening. This was dealt with by standardizing our screening process, which appears to be working well.

Another problem that arose is the very high proportion of Native Americans in the sample populations. We decided to stratify the sample by ethnicity, using the overall population proportion as criteria for the sample (39% Native Americans). In this way, we can be assured of adequate representativeness from the two major groups of clients in the population.

Procedures for assessment and treatment planning were implemented in late September, and were in place within 30 days. Clients are randomly assigned to case managers, who then do a comprehensive assessment using the ASI as cornerstone. In addition, county policy requires that all clients must be assessed in 15 areas of life. A treatment plan is completed within 30 days, and is reassessed every 6 months.

Interventions involve frequent contact, non-judgemental support, and specific focus on improving housing and establishing abstinence or reduced drinking. The team appears to be very successful in keeping contact with clients, and clients seem appreciative. A standardized system for classifying and treating clients using clinical "tiers" described earlier, has been implemented. The team is now assessing its feasibility and altering it as needed. Weekend coverage is provided, with one counselor seeing any clients in ARC. Team function is monitored closely through daily contact with the unit supervisor and project director. The PI and Evaluation

Director meet with the Project Director weekly or more frequently to monitor the team's effectiveness and to solve problems. The following case vignette illustrates how ICM actually works.

CTCPI staff attempted to commit a client to treatment to shelter him from the Minnesota winter. The client was 73 years old, and legendary to the system. The Probate Court refused to grant this commitment and the client was told he could leave. However, the client was in shirt sleeves and the outside temperature was minus two degrees with a wind chill.

The client said, "I can get back to the building where my coat is, I've been in plenty of cold in my life." (Client's coat was 1.5 miles away.) His case manager, Steve, said, "No, it's below zero, we'll get a ride for you."

An outside party, an attorney, said, "The son of a . . . just beat you in court, let the . . . walk and find out just where he's at."

The client's case manager and the project director insisted that the judge order the sheriff to transport the client to where his coat was located. She did so order.

Housing

Efforts in housing have taken place on parallel levels of system and client. On the system level, we have been very active in advocating for more, and more appropriate housing for our clients. Lack of housing is the single most difficult barrier to overcome for most of them. The Project Director appeared before the City Council, and was able to obtain an exception from a moratorium on granting conditional use permits for projects such as half-way houses. We have had ongoing discussions with Catholic Charities about establishing another residence specifically for CPIs in Hennepin County (they have one in Ramsey County). We have supported the law allowing representative payee status for economic assistance payments. This will allow us to vendor-pay a housing vendor on behalf of a client.

Case managers also have routinely found housing, provided transportation, and then accompanied their clients to the dwelling and assisted them in making suitable arrangements. They have advocated for them with landlords and agencies. Because of this activity, there have been striking improvements in housing for most of the clients, in spite of the housing shortage. Individual case managers have been networking with other care providers, as they serve their clients. Housing and economic assistance constitute the bulk of their interactions. However, as time goes on, they are increasingly becoming aware of the need to become involved with a much more informal network of supporters, both public and private. This informal network is more difficult to interact with, because of its shifting, informal nature, high staff turnover, and abrupt changes in their mission in order to respond to client needs. Case managers are concentrating their efforts on linking with both formal and informal systems.

OUTCOME EVALUATION

Client Selection and Grouping

Based on an examination of ARC records, a pool of potential clients who meet selection criteria (more than 15 ARC admissions and male), was created and randomized into three comparison groups; ICM, NICM and EC. ARC admissions are screened to find individuals in the subject pool. If an individual on the list is discovered to be in the ARC, he is screened to determine if he is homeless. If he is, and if he agrees to participate, he is entered into his pre-assigned clinical program. (Follow-up information that is not dependent on interview data is obtained for those who refuse to participate to assess sample bias.)

The intensive case management group (ICM) receives the most intensive level of care as described earlier. To date, 56 clients have been selected.

The non-intensive case management group (NICM) consists of up to 150 homeless clients with alcohol problems. (Thus far, 109 individuals have been recruited.) They are served by three case managers funded by Health Care for the Homeless. These case managers are supervised by a unit supervisor in an existing program within the program center managed by the Principal Investigator. The model of case management is relatively similar in philosophy to that of the ICM program, but the higher caseload makes it impossible to carry out many of the innovative aspects of intensive case management. Case managers spend most of their time in their offices, and less time in client search or outside agency coordination.

The episodic care (EC) control group is so named because the model of treatment that was extant over the last few years provided episodic evaluation and referral of clients, depending on their presence or absence in detox. While there was a familiarity with certain clients that developed over the years, no actual case management occurred. For example, there was no attempt to coordinate the various service elements, and interventions were primarily focused on alcoholism. A sample of 85-100 clients will be selected for this group; 20 have been selected thus far.

Clients are being evaluated through the use of self-reports of their perceptions of their medical, chemical and psychological status, and through tracking utilization and expense of various services provided within the county. The goal is to assess cost efficacy as well as clinical efficacy.

Sample Characteristics

Clinical and demographic sample characteristics are summarized in Table 1. We had noted that the most severely disordered clients were selected first, because of frequent ARC admissions. In order to control for this effect, we matched groups by order of program entry. Since the NICM group was about twice as large as the ICM group, that meant that we compared the first half of the NICM group admitted (Group 1) to the ICM group. The second group of NICM subjects admitted (Group 2) will be compared with other ICM subjects as more are added to that group. Significant differences between NICM Groups 1 and 2 are apparent in racial composition and past ARC use. While the ICM group has more past ARC use, the difference is not statistically significant, and its racial composition is similar to NICM/G1. Race was not significantly related to past ARC use in any single group, in the NICM group as a whole or across ICM and NICM groups.

Analysis of the distribution of ARC admits across groups (not shown) indicates that there are more of the very severe cases in the

Table 1. Characteristics of Intensive (ICM) and Nonintensive (NICM) Case Management and Episodic Care (EC) Groups

	ICM (N=55)		NICM/G1* (n=56)		NICM/G2* (N=53)		EC (N=20)	
	M	(SD)	M	(SD)	M	(SD)	M	(SD)
Age	43.3	(10.3)	41.9	(10.3)	42.4	(9.7)	37.5	(10.3)
ARC Admits (Lifetime)	113.3	(13.3)	97.9	(92.9)	57.6**	(69.2)	96.8	(93.1)
ARC Admits (Past Year)	21.3	(21.4)	15.9	(10.2)	10.8	(10.7)	17.6	(11.5)
Months in Prgm	4.9	(0.9)	9.4	(0.8)	5.9	(1.8)	7.2	(2.3)
ASI Composite Scores			(Combined NICM groups)					
Medical	.389	(.315)	.293	(.022)				
Alcohol	.574	(.208)	.491	(.233)				
Drug	.016	(.061)	.017	(.045)				
Psych	.144	(.183)	.106	(.196)				
Race (In Percent)								
Native Am	58		50		36		75	
Black/Hisp	15		18		4		10	
Caucasian	27		32		60		15	

*The NICM groups is subdivided into the first 56 clients admitted to the program (G1) and the next 53 (G2).

** $P < .05$

ICM group than in NICM/Gl. These differences are not statistically significant, probably because a few outliers tend to distort the data, especially in the ICM group. Thus, it makes sense to consider removing these from some analyses, especially those heavily dependent on measures of central tendency. All in all, it appears that there are no significant differences between ICM and NICM clients, provided order of program entry is taken into account.

Initial Outcome Results

Data available for analysis at this time are shown in Table 2. The outcome variable related to ARC admits is average ARC admits/ month, while in the program (i.e., the total number of ARC admits since program entry is divided by the number of months since program entry). All groups have shown an increase in the mean number of admits/month, but this is only significant in the two NICM groups. Examination of the medians (not shown), however, sug-

Table 2. Initial Results in Some Outcome Measures Across Groups

	ICM (N=55)		NICM/G1* (n=56)		NICM/G2* (N=53)		EC (N=20)	
	M	(SD)	M	(SD)	M	(SD)	M	(SD)
ARC Admits/mo Year prior to Program Entry	1.8	(1.9)	1.3	(0.8)	0.9	(0.9)*	2.5	(1.3)
ARC Admits/mo Since program Entry	2.2	(2.3)	1.9	(1.5)^	1.4	(1.5)^*	2.7	(1.6)
Ratings** of Improvement Since Entry			(Combined NICM groups)					
Drinking	3.8	(1.1)			3.3	(1.1)		
Housing	3.6	(0.9)			3.6	(1.2)		
Overall	3.6	(1.1)			3.3	(1.2)		
Percent with Improvement in at Least 2 of 3 Categories	43		36					
Dropouts(%)	2		20					

* Difference between NICM Groups 1 and 2 significant by t-test, p<.05

^ Difference between year prior and current year significant by paired-sample t-test, p<.05.

** Scale 1=a lot worse, 2=a little worse, 3=unchanged, 4=a little better, 5= a lot better. Time frame for rating: past 30 days compared to entry.

gested that the mean values may again be distorted by outliers. The same order of relationship exists among the three groups as in Total and Year prior ARC admits, but in this case, there are no significant differences. All three groups appear to be utilizing detox at a similar rate since program entry.

The difference between ICM and NICM on dropout rates (Table 2) approaches significance. Not shown are data from other county detox centers and the detox center in Ramsey County (St. Paul). These data show that relatively few project subjects utilize these services. The ones who do tend not to be using the Hennepin County ARC.

In order to obtain clinical information that would not necessarily appear in any of our measures, we constructed a simple rating scale for case managers to use to rate their clients' global progress in the areas of drinking, overall functioning and housing. The instrument asks each case manager to rate each client in the three areas. In each area, the rating is that the client's function in that area is 1 – "a lot worse," 2 – "a little worse," 3 – "unchanged," 4 – "a little better," 5 – "a lot better." The time frame is the last 30 days, as compared to an earlier period (such as program entry, the last rating, etc.)

Initial results of the global ratings in the ICM and NICM groups are shown in Table 2. A majority of both groups are rated as improved over baseline in each area, especially housing. Substantial minorities are rated as improved in 2 out of 3 areas.

DISCUSSION

Our experience suggests that it is feasible to implement a program of intensive case management (ICM) for the long-term community treatment of homeless chronic public inebriates (CPIs). Barriers encountered here included staff turnover, resistance of some staff within our agency, stigmatization of the clientele, and a severe shortage of low-income housing. Clear support by the administration of our agency has been essential to the successful implementation of the project.

Within our population of CPIs, there appears to be a gradient of severity, such that the first 150 out of 600 are much more severely impaired. Native Americans are disproportionately represented in this most severe group, for reasons that are not clear. A question of some urgency is why Native Americans are utilizing ARC so much, and other agencies so little. We are currently implementing an ethnographic study to examine this issue in more depth.

All three comparison groups are showing increased ARC utilization during the current year, compared to the year prior. This is not unexpected, given changes in the Chemical Health Division policy towards CPIs in the last year. An analysis of the cost-effectiveness of commitment to residential primary chemical dependency treatment by the county suggested that little or no reduction in ARC admissions was obtained with costly procedures and treatment. Consequently, CPIs are no longer being committed to treatment unless there are very clear indications of probable improvement (e.g., motivation, prior response, etc.). Many of the most serious CPIs spent a significant amount of time in a residential facility in the year prior to program entry, but that has since ceased.

At about the same time, ARC began discharging known clients earlier, in order to clear beds more rapidly. This has led to an increase in turnover, and an increase in number of admissions (perhaps with some reduction in length of stay) for some high users of ARC. Thus, we expected ARC admissions to rise. At this point, they do not seem to be rising or falling more rapidly in one group than the next.

The results of the global outcome ratings by the case managers are encouraging, and may indicate early improvement that will later result in changes in system utilization. The only indication of differences between case management groups at this point is the difference in dropout rates. If this difference in rate of dropout increases over time, as expected, then that alone may result in differences in outcome.

The dropout rates were rather low, compared to projections. We also found very little utilization of other county detox facilities, or by the detox facility in an adjacent county. This runs counter to expectations, and suggests that CPIs may be more stable and less transient than previously thought.

REFERENCES

Annis, H.M., Smart, R.G. (1976). Arrests, readmissions and treatment following release from detoxification centers. *J Stud Alcohol*, 39, 1276-1283.

Ashley, M.J., Olin, J.S., LeRiche, W.H., Kornaczewski, A., Schmidt, W., Ranking, J.G. (1983). Skid row alcoholism: A distinct sociomedical entity. *Arch Int Med*, 136, 272-278.

Baker, F.M. (1985). ER 'capture' of the skid-row alcoholic. *Gen Hosp Psych*, 7, 138-143.

Bassuk, E.L., Rubin, L., Alison, L. (1984). Is homelessness a mental health problem? *Am J Psychiatry*, 141, 1546-1550.

Blower, C. (1978). Alcoholism and derelicts in the inner metropolitan region of Sydney, *Med J Austr*, 1, 210-211.

Blumberg, L.U., Shipley, T.E., Moor, J.O. (1971). The skid row man and the skid row status community, *OJ Stud Alc*, 32, 909-941.

Cohen, C.I., Sokolovsky, J. (1983). Toward a concept of homelessness among aged men, *J Gerontology*, 38, 81-89.

Combs-Orme, T., Taylor, J.R., Rovins, J.N., Holmes, S.J. (1983). Differential mortality among alcoholics by sample site, *AJPH*, 73, 900-903.

Ditman, K.S., Crawford, G.G., Forgy, E.W., Moskowitz, H., MacAndrew, C. (1967). A controlled experiment on the use of court probation for drunk arrests, *Amer J Psych*, 124, 160-167.

Finn, P. (1985). Decriminalization of public drunkenness: Response of the health care system, *J Stud Alc*, 46, 7-23.

Kurtz, N.R., Regier, M. (1975). The uniform alcoholism and intoxication treatment act. The compromising process of social policy formulation, *J Stud Alc* 36, 1421-1441.

Langsley, D.G. (1985). Community psychiatry, in Kaplan, H.I., and Sadock, B.J., eds., *Comprehensive Textbook of Psychiatry*, Baltimore, Williams and Wilkins.

Lovald, K., Stub, H.R. (1968). The revolving door: Reactions of chronic drunkenness offenders to court sanctions, *J Crim Law*, 59, 525-530.

McIntosh, I.D. (1982). Alcohol-related disabilities in general hospital patients: A critical assessment of the evidence, *Int J Addic*, 17, 609-639.

Miller, P.M. (1975). A behavioral intervention program for chronic public drunkenness offenders, *Arch Gen Psych*, 32, 915-918.

Moos, R.H., Mehren, B., Moos, B.S. (1978). Evaluation of a salvation army alcoholism treatment program, *J Stud Alc*, 39, 1267-1275.

Myerson, D.J., Mayer, J. (1966). Origins, treatment, and density of skid-row alcoholic men, *NEJM*, 275, 419-425.

Neuner, R., Schultz, D. (1986). Borrow Me A Quarter: A Study of the Feasibility of the Prepaid Case-Management System for the Chronic Recidivist Alcoholic, St. Paul, Minnesota Institute of Public Health.

Ogbourne, A., Collier, D. (1979). A rehabilitation programme with a controlled drinking option, *Int J Soc Psychiatry*, 25, 47-55.

Pittman, D.J., (1974). Interaction between skid row people and law enforcement and health professionals, *Addict Dis*, 1, 369-388.

Pratt, A.D. (1976). A mandatory treatment program for skid row alcoholics; its implication for the uniform alcoholism and intoxication treatment act, *J Stud Alc*, 36, 166-170.

Reinke, B., Greenley, J.R. (1986). Organizational analysis of three community support program models, *Hosp Comm Psych*, 37, 624-629.

Richman, A., Neumann, B. (1984). Breaking the 'detox-loop' for alcoholics with social detoxification, *Drug Alc Depen*, 13, 65-73.

Rosenberg, C.M., Liftik, J. (1976). Use of coercion in the outpatient treatment of alcoholism, *J Stud Alc*, 37, 58-65.

Roth, D., Bean, J. (1985). Alcohol problems and homelessness: Findings from the Ohio study, *Alc Health Res World*, Wtr 1985/6, pp 14-15.

Schwartzburg, M.S., Schwartz, A. (1976). A five-year study of brief hospitalization, *Am J. Psych* 133, 922-924.

Stein, L.I., Test, M.A. (1980). Alternative to mental hospital treatment I: Conceptual model, treatment program, and clinical evaluation, *Arch Gen Psych*, 37, 392-397.

Test, M.A. (1979). Continuity of care in community treatment, in Stein, L.I., ed., *Community Support Systems for the Long-term Patient*, San Francisco, Jossey-Bass, pp 15-24.

Weisbrod, B.A., Test, M.A., Stein, L.I. (1980). Alternative to mental hospital treatment II: Economic benefit-cost analysis, *Arch Gen Psych*, 37, 400-498.

Wells, J.E. (1985). Recurrent alcoholism: Readmissions for treatment for alcoholism, *NZ Med J*, 98, 500-503.

Woogh, C.M. (1986). A cohort through the revolving door, *Can J Psychiatry*, 31, 214-221.

Zimberg, S. (1974). Evaluation of alcoholism treatment in Harlem, *QJ Stud Alc*, 35, 550-557.

Outreach and Engagement for Homeless Women at Risk of Alcoholism

Sylvia Ridlen, PhD
Yvonne Asamoah, PhD
Helen G. Edwards, MPH
Rita Zimmer, MPH

Women with children represent a relatively new but growing homeless population. New York City, for example, temporarily houses some 5,000 such families in public and private shelters and "welfare hotels" (NYC Human Resources Administration, 1987). Countless more families are at imminent risk of homelessness because they are living doubled up with friends or family, live in buildings which do not meet fire safety standards, or face eviction.

Alcohol use among the homeless is considerable with alcohol abuse and alcoholism estimated at 3-6 times greater than in the general population (Lubran, 1987). However, it is far from clear that the traditional model of alcoholism as a progressive disease leading to problems (like homelessness) accurately describes the situation for homeless women. Rather, women may drink as a way to cope with their problems.

The issue is further confused by traditional alcoholism treatment's relative ineffectiveness with women. For example, the confrontational techniques often used for male compulsory treatment may frighten women or encourage passive responses. Further, tra-

Sylvia Ridlen is Program Evaluator, Yvonne Asamoah is Research Consultant, Helen G. Edwards is Research Associate, and Rita Zimmer is Principal Investigator and Executive Director, Women In Need, 410 W. 40th Street, New York, NY 10018.

99

ditional treatment models give little consideration to women's on-going family responsibilities, which usually do not stop while they are in treatment. Lastly, the special cultural, ethnic and racial characteristics of the adult hotel population as these affect alcohol treatment service delivery have been hardly explored.

THE SETTING

Women In Need, Inc., is a private nonprofit multi-service agency created in 1982 in response to a lack of appropriate services for homeless women and their children in New York City. It has grown rapidly because of great need and community support. The organization runs a number of small shelters as well as several programs to serve hotel families. Among its several programs is an outpatient alcohol clinic.

The alcohol clinic was funded in 1987 by the New York City Department of Mental Health, Mental Retardation and Alcohol Services, and is licensed by the New York State Division of Alcoholism. State regulations and funding priorities which reflected a traditional alcoholism treatment model limited the provision of outreach and engagement services considered most relevant to homeless women. As a result the clinic had limited success in attracting and engaging homeless women in its first year of operation. The National Institute on Alcohol Abuse and Alcoholism Community Demonstration Project provided the opportunity to design a project which focuses on providing outreach, engagement and support services to homeless women (mostly minority) with alcohol problems.

PROJECT DESCRIPTION

Funded for two years beginning in September 1988, the Project is designed to provide outreach, engagement and support services to a population of homeless females, mostly Black and Hispanic, who live in two Manhattan "welfare hotels." Specifically, the project offers assistance with immediate problems, provides referrals, follow-up and advocacy. Services include: acupuncture, employment assistance, housing relocation, GED/literacy, respite child care and alcoholism treatment services.

Goals

1. Attract homeless alcohol abusing women into treatment
2. Develop an effective outreach/engagement model for alcohol abusing homeless women with children
3. Design and implement an outreach/engagement model that is relevant to racial, cultural and economic diversity of the target population
4. Improve access to services which support sobriety and enhance the quality of life of homeless females

Objectives

1. Increase the number of homeless women utilizing the alcohol clinic
2. Increase access to programs and personnel supportive of sobriety for women and children
3. Develop an inservice training model which increases knowledge and sensitivity to the impact of race, culture and class on values, choices and decision making

STRUCTURE OF SERVICE DELIVERY/ PROJECT IMPLEMENTATION

The core of the project's service delivery emanates from two outreach teams (one is housed in each hotel). Each team includes a team leader, who has both direct service and team supervisory responsibilities, an outreach counselor (with expertise in alcoholism counseling) and an outreach worker. Outreach counselors do much of the initial assessment, while outreach workers stress the outreach, rapport-building, and supportive concrete service activities (like escorting clients to appointments). Initial outreach efforts include providing project literature and a general explanation of the project's services. For safety purposes, team members generally work in pairs when knocking on hotel doors and seeing clients away from the team office.

Women who express interest in obtaining services are asked to participate in an initial assessment interview which usually lasts about an hour. This interview is conducted by a team member, and is based on McLelland's (1980) Addiction Severity Index (ASI). The original ASI was modified and expanded to better fit our homeless female population. This expanded ASI interview provides the basis for assessing legal, family and social relationships, drug and alcohol use, medical, psychiatric, and employment/economic functioning. Relevant social history, demographic and other data are also obtained. Written informed consent to use the interview data for research purposes is obtained before the interview is begun. Based on this initial assessment interview and a woman's expressed interests, plans are made and referrals initiated. At the point when women are clearly connected to services, the outreach team continues to be involved by providing case management services.

OTHER PROJECT SERVICES

Acupuncture is available to women in conjunction with alcohol treatment, for stress, or other conditions. Acupuncture is a service new to Women In Need and was initiated for this project.

Housing assistance has been successfully offered by Women In Need to its shelter residents for several years. Housing specialists provide assistance negotiating the application process for public housing programs and with private landlords with whom relationships have been cultivated. Women's housing needs are assessed, and a match is sought with available apartments.

Once a woman is linked with an apartment, she is then given essential information about her new neighborhood in preparation for moving (e.g., location and telephone number of utilities, schools, and other essential services) and is provided with household necessities and moving assistance. Recently, a series of six workshops was begun to educate women about topics ranging from tenants' rights to apartment interviews and budgeting. This training is expected to facilitate client transition into permanent housing. After relocation to permanent housing, women are followed for several months and are encouraged to contact the housing program in the event of problems at any time.

Respite child care for children six months to six years of age is available. In addition, a child care coordinator makes temporary housing arrangements for children whose mothers need inpatient detoxification. This coordinator works cooperatively with public and private child care agencies so women in need of short-term child care are assured that it will indeed be short-term. (In the past, women have resisted temporary foster placement through the city's child protective services agency, fearing they would have difficulty regaining custody of their children.)

An education specialist provides assessment of educational needs, individual tutoring, and group classes to prepare women for the high school general equivalency diploma (GED) test. When special needs are evident, the educational specialist tries to make appropriate referrals. An employment specialist is also available part-time. This specialist links available jobs with suitable applicants. Training in job readiness skills and supportive counselling are also provided.

The alcohol clinic accepts referrals from the NIAAA project. Individual and group counseling are provided six days a week. Breathalyser and urine tests are randomly conducted on a regular basis and provide tangible evidence to clients and staff of alcohol consumption.

ORGANIZATIONAL CONTEXT

The outreach and engagement project is very complex, and involves a number of interrelated components and services. The housing and child care project components are located in pre-existing Women In Need programs, but the staff are closely identified with the project. This situation poses special challenges for staff and Women In Need program administration as well as the project director. Other components represent services new to the Women In Need organization, which must learn to relate to these services as part of the agency, even though the services may be unavailable to most Women In Need clients.

The host organization (Women In Need) within which and through which services are provided, ultimately plays a major part in the successful implementation of the project. Women In Need is an organization which has undergone phenomenally, even boom, rapid growth. The usual result of such rapid growth in organizations is a lag in infrastructure capacity and difficulties in incorporating and integrating all new staff and programs promptly into the organizational identity and culture.

The temporary nature of this project may be cause for the organization to resist fully accepting project staff. In boom towns, for example, "newcomers" often find it very difficult to join in or be accepted in the community; they are blamed for the community's growing pains, stresses and problems, and viewed as temporary residents who are likely to move on soon. Similarly, newcomers often hesitate to invest emotionally in a community where they don't feel welcome and perhaps also expect to leave soon.

Women In Need seems better able to cope with such problems in some ways than most organizations. Perhaps innovative programs can be best accommodated by existing organizations that are not rigidly bound by established procedures and traditions. At Women In Need everyone is relatively new. Also, the organization's culture and philosophy are founded on respect and inclusion of staff and clients.

On the other hand, the programs of Women In Need are scattered among three boroughs, so organizational and staff identity are difficult to establish and maintain in the first place. Space has been the infrastructure problem that has been most constant and problematic in the face of rapid growth. In mid-Manhattan, suitable space that is also affordable is nearly impossible to find in a timely fashion. The funding of the demonstration project meant that for the first nine months of the project, the organization's administrative offices and support services were even more over-crowded than before. This contributed to some strains between project staff and the organization.

In retrospect, it seems that allowing five months for project start-up was insufficient. Staff and organization familiarity with one another still need strengthening. Furthermore, the complexity of the project itself meant that establishing administrative policy, and decision making structures took time. Also, project staff required extensive orientation to the project. A longer start-up phase might have allowed for the establishment of a larger applicant pool for staff positions.

The decision to use clinical data and records for research purposes required special training and several revisions of data collection forms and procedures. Staff, who are service-oriented, had to learn to take the extra steps of translating clinical records into quantifiable categories and terms.

The structure, staff, data collection instruments, and office equipment and supplies are mostly now in place; four months after service delivery began. One exception is that a Spanish-speaking team member could not be found, although it was a high priority to hire at least one bilingual team member. A translator has recently been hired, and should enhance the efficiency of helping clients complete forms and interviews and make essential contacts with other service providers. The lack of bilingual staff seems all the more significant in that nearly 40% of the clients served to date are Hispanic.

The outreach teams and other staff have had a unique training program which has proved essential for several reasons. The team members have a great deal of enthusiasm and optimism, and the training has been the main channel for converting initial anxiety and motivation into purposeful helping.

Early training sessions included development of skills and provision of information connected with homelessness, team building, engagement, the nature of outreach work, referral resources in each hotel community, and the need for and process of functional assessment. Later training sessions have focused on specific content related to substance abuse and actual assessment. Ongoing training seems necessary to enable the teams to integrate outreach work and service delivery, and to begin to address significant clinical issues with this population.

The teams have now reached a level of comfort with various project service components and the data collection and recording procedures. Reaching this point was not easy for reasons already discussed and because of the intensity and difficulties inherent in working with homeless families and substance abuse problems, in a society that devalues such clients. Recognition of the difficult nature of outreach work with this population and in the hotel setting is essential to sustain staff morale and prevent burnout.

EVALUATION

Because the project is for research demonstration, it is important that it be fully evaluated and documented. Over 25% of the total budget is devoted to research. The evaluation includes process and outcome components.

The evaluation is designed to accomplish the following objectives:

1. determine the relative effectiveness of each of the project's component programs in relation to alcohol treatment
2. document program component utilization rates and patterns
3. describe and document in detail project activities, deployment of resources, and attainment of project objectives
4. describe the target and clinic populations
5. document staff and client experiences and perceptions in such a manner that program modifications and refinements can be made when indicated

The process evaluation relies on both qualitative and quantitative information. Quantitative data include utilization, demographic, and activity data. Qualitative data are derived from periodic interviews with project staff, informal contacts with other service delivery staff in the hotels, hotel residents and from non-participant (but unconcealed) observation in the hotels and the streets adjacent to them. Information is also drawn from the written minutes of staff and administrative meetings and staff training sessions.

Follow-up interviews of staff and clients after two months of service and again at 6 month intervals will help refine the service components of the project and the quantitative data collection by identifying gaps, inefficiencies, confusion, or redundancies. Qualitative interview data often provide information and insights not easily obtained through quantitative methods. Such data also provide a rough reliability and validity check of the quantitative analysis and its interpretation.

The first round of staff interviews was done between February 1st and April 20th, 1989, shortly after outreach and other services began (the first five months of the project were devoted to start-up). Administrative, research, and direct service delivery staff were all interviewed as were selected alcohol clinic staff. Perceptions of the project's early functioning, problems, and strengths by those most intimately involved have been extremely important for making needed adjustments and revisions. Further, staff's observations and perceptions of clients provide valuable insights to guide analysis of service effectiveness and impact.

Interviews with clients who have been with the project at least two months are just beginning, and will be repeated at six month intervals. These client interviews are not required, but we hope most women will agree to be interviewed. The interviews are intended to assess the long-term relevance of project component services, changes in needs, priorities, and client perceptions as management of alcohol problems and quality of life improve. Clients' interviews will also provide valuable and critical information on their motivation, elaboration of their perceived needs and priorities, and their perceptions of the accessibility and relevance of staff and service. These data are essential if the outreach and engagement project is to succeed.

The efficacy of the project is not likely to become clear until services have been available for at least six months. In the next few months, staff and clients will gain familiarity and comfort with services and their utilization. The plan of analysis for utilization and client outcome data includes time series analysis and repeated measures tests. Levels of alcohol consumption and changes in employment, educational level, and housing status will be assessed.

PRELIMINARY RESULTS

Demographics. After three months of outreach, 49 women have requested services and subsequently become clients of the project. Forty-three women are currently active, meaning they have had some contact with either the outreach team or other project component staff within the last six weeks. The six inactive clients remain eligible for services.

The age of these 49 women range from 19 to 44 years. Thirty-five percent are aged 18-24, fifty-one percent are 25-34 and the remaining fourteen percent are 35-44 years of age. There appears to be an over-representation of Hispanics in the present client population, compared to the general hotel population. Based on estimates of hotel service providers (Special Services for Children and Crisis Intervention Services Staff), the general hotel population is 70% black, 25% Hispanic and 5% other. However, 39% of the project's clients are Hispanic, 59% are black, and 2% fall into the "other" category.

Service Requests and Referrals. The service most often requested is housing assistance. As shown in Table 1, thirty of the 43 active clients have asked to see the housing specialist. Currently, two of these women have been tentatively linked to permanent housing through Women In Need. Two others have been relocated through other efforts.

The second most requested service is GED/education, with 19 women asking for this service. Employment services have been requested by 10 clients. One of these women recently started a new job as a result of her involvement with the project. Eleven women have requested a referral to the alcoholism clinic and 4 women asked to see the acupuncturist.

Table 1. Services Requested and Offered

Service Component	Number of Requests	Number of Offers
Housing Assistance	30	23
GED/Education	19	12
Employment	10	9
Child Care	12	8
Acupuncture	4	10
Alcoholism Clinic	11	14

Besides the women's own requests, Table 1 also shows the actual offers of services made by teams after their initial assessment was completed. Some women who requested housing assistance have not yet been offered those services. However, services at the alcohol clinic and acupuncture were offered to more women than were requested.

CONCLUSION

An innovative program tailored to meet the needs of homeless, minority women in welfare hotels is providing valuable insights into the needs of such a population and appropriate models of service delivery. Initial responses have been greater and much faster than expected. While outreach and engagement with street people is often slow work, hotel women have responded eagerly and show good motivation to use services which they believe will improve their circumstances. The effects of these supportive services on alcohol consumption and treatment are of central interest in this project.

REFERENCES

Housing Resources Administration (October, 1987) *Five Year Plan for Housing Homeless Families*. City of New York.
Lubran, B.G. (Spring, 1987) Alcohol-related problems among the homeless: NIAAA's response. *Alcohol Health and Research World*, 4-6, 73.
McLellan, A.T., Luborsky, L., and Woody, G.E. (1980) An improved evaluation instrument for substance abuse patients: The Addiction Severity Index. *Journal of Nervous and Mental Diseases*, 168: 26-33.

Alameda County Department of Alcohol and Drug Programs Comprehensive Homeless Alcohol Recovery Services (CHARS)

Robert W. Bennett, MA
Hazel L. Weiss, MA
Barbara R. West, PhD

Comprehensive approaches to the problems of homelessness, alcohol, and other drugs emerged as a result of three historical developments. The first is the changing face of homelessness in America and accompanying slow disappearance of the typical skid row alcoholic, as he was traditionally defined, from the landscape of American cities. Fiercely independent, white, male, and committed to alcohol as the only drug of choice, it was easy to attribute the causes of his many problems to individual pathology: a sick spirit enslaved by the demon alcohol, or a chemical dependent in need of medical treatment. The perspective that alcohol and other drug problems are caused by pathologies at the individual level is naturally accompanied by the view that their amelioration is best approached by providing them with personal spiritual, physical, or psychological treatment. As Piliavin (1989) reminds us, "remedies follow the themes of the explanations."

Today's research literature confirms what long-term providers in the alcohol field have experienced in their own work, that the pro-

Robert W. Bennett is affiliated with Resource Development Associates. Hazel L. Weiss is associated with the Alameda County Department of Alcohol and Drug Programs, 499 Fifth Street, Oakland, CA 94607. Barbara R. West is affiliated with the Pacific Institute for Research and Evaluation.

file of homelessness has changed substantially and along with it, the profile of individuals seen in both detox and residential recovery programs. Increasingly, they are younger poly-drug users from minority communities; alcohol is rarely their only drug of choice. The factors placing young people at risk of both drug problems and delinquency have been found to cluster. Hawkins et al. (1986) present a strong case for certain indicators as reliable covariants of both drug problems and delinquency. These include parent/sibling drug use and criminal behavior; poor and inconsistent family management practices; the presence of family conflict; social deprivation; school failure and/or drop out; a peer group with many of the same attributes. These findings point to causal agency in social groups, in families, peer groups, formal organizations such as schools, and in communities where life is defined by the absence of opportunities for success in legitimate pursuits.

Historical changes in the characteristics of homeless people with alcohol and other drug problems, well-documented by Stark (1987) and Garrett (1989), have required changing paradigms and their policy implications, not to exclude the focus on individuals, but rather to expand the focus to include environmental and system issues. A recent study of "Mental Health, Alcohol and Drug Use, and Criminal History Among Homeless Adults," found that "many homeless adults have an overwhelming set of social, mental health, criminal, alcohol, and drug problems," suggesting to the authors that diverse systems of care are needed, "aimed at various subgroups of the homeless," (Gelberg et al., 1988). Wright and Weber (1988) documented incredible deprivation among homeless individuals, many of whom fail to qualify for any financial benefits.

Massive increases in the sheer number of homeless individuals is the second historical development to prompt re-examination of individual level theories of pathology and remediation. Arguing that "the roots of marginality . . . lie in the basic needs-meeting mechanisms of society, affordable housing in particular," Kaufman (1989) challenges the view that homelessness is a problem of "troubled — and troublesome — individuals." A program addressing the problems of the homeless at a more systemic level might require:

Drastic increases in low cost housing, improvements in the level of welfare payments, better community-based services for the deinstitutionalized mentally ill, and increased institutional space and services for those among the mentally ill, unable to sustain community life. And finally for that residual group of individuals not aided by these other programs, shelters must be built which provide "adequate" food, space, privacy and safety. (Piliavin, 1989)

The third process contributing to the evolution of comprehensive approaches involves lessons learned from the research literature on prevention. In the Handbook for Prevention Evaluation (1983) NIDA identified four modalities of primary drug abuse prevention: information, education, alternatives, and intervention. To these NIAAA added environmental change programs and social policy change. Moskowitz (1984) critically reviewed the effects of programs and policies in reducing the incidence of alcohol problems and concluded that, "the research generally supported the efficacy of three alcohol-specific policies: raising the minimum legal drinking age to 21, increasing alcohol taxes and increasing the enforcement of drinking-driving laws." He also concluded that various environmental safety measures reduce the incidence and severity of alcohol-related trauma. In contrast, little evidence was found to support the efficacy of primary prevention programs. A systems perspective of prevention suggests, however, that prevention programs could, "become more efficacious after widespread adoption of prevention policies that lead to shifts in social norms regarding use of beverage alcohol."

A U.S. Department of Education/U.S. Department of Health and Human Services (1987) report to the Congress on the nature and effectiveness of federal, state, and local programs of drug prevention summarized their findings as follows:

(1) The causes of substance abuse include factors at all levels of society—the individual, family, peer group, schools, community, and the larger social environment; (2) traditionally, most prevention programs have focused only on the individual

in an attempt to remedy perceived deficiencies of knowledge, coping skills, or behavior; more recently, prevention has begun to address the individual within the context of peers, families, schools, and communities; (3) comprehensive programs that address a number of factors influencing drug use are likely to hold the most promise of prevention; and (4) prevention efforts that focus on only one or two factors are unlikely to be successful.

The Alameda County Department of Alcohol and Drug Programs (DADP) developed its Comprehensive Homeless Alcohol Recovery Services (CHARS) program based on a model which reflects this research and its policy implications. This model posits a continual interaction between five levels of society which can encourage or inhibit drinking and drug use. These levels include; (1) the larger legal and cultural environment, (2) the community environment, (3) the family and workplace environment, (4) immediate drinking environments, and (5) individual factors. Social change activities may be directed at any level and, if successful, impact all the others. Since alcoholism, seen in its broadest context, is a community illness, those individuals who are physiologically addicted to the drug represent only a part of the full scope and severity of alcohol problems in the United States. (See Figure 1.)

Therefore, our responses to alcohol problems must be extended beyond the provision of recovery opportunities for the increasing number of individuals who may be considered alcoholic. Efforts must be made to reduce the incidence of all alcohol problems at the family, societal, and public policy levels.

Alcohol problems occur as a result of the interaction of many factors: and require a complex solution — a solution which encompasses intervention at the individual, family, and societal levels and which is based on the combined efforts of many segments of our society. Factors contributing to alcohol problems include attitudes toward the role of alcohol in our society as reflected in the media, the manner in which alcohol beverages are advertised and otherwise marketed, public policies regarding availability of the drug, and social values regarding

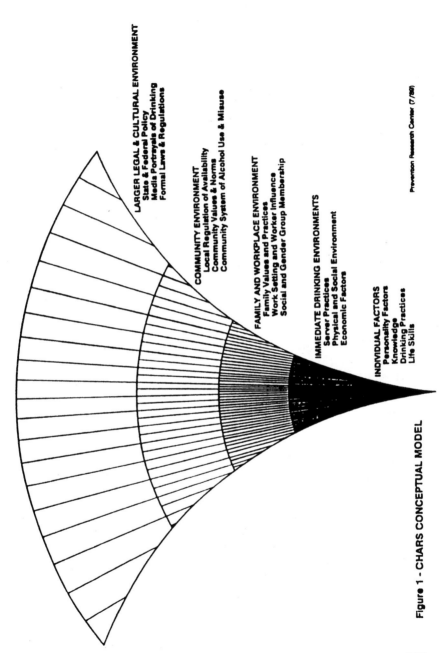

LARGER LEGAL & CULTURAL ENVIRONMENT
State & Federal Policy
Media Portrayals of Drinking
Formal Laws & Regulations

COMMUNITY ENVIRONMENT
Local Regulation of Availability
Community Values & Norms
Community System of Alcohol Use & Misuse

FAMILY AND WORKPLACE ENVIRONMENT
Family Values and Practices
Work Setting and Worker Influence
Social and Gender Group Membership

IMMEDIATE DRINKING ENVIRONMENTS
Server Practices
Physical and Social Environment
Economic Factors

INDIVIDUAL FACTORS
Personality Factors
Knowledge
Drinking Practices
Life Skills

Prevention Research Center (7/89)

Figure 1 - CHARS CONCEPTUAL MODEL

115

the nature and use of the drug. (1988-89 Alameda County Plan for the Prevention of Alcohol Related Problems)

PROGRAM DESCRIPTION

In Alameda County, over 6,000 homeless people — the majority of whom are women and their young children — have been turned away every month from a 413 bed shelter system already filled to capacity. Additional numbers of homeless people — difficult to count, yet nonetheless present — reside under freeways, in abandoned buildings, in cars, parks, and doorways.

With this large and rapidly growing homeless population, Alameda County has been at the forefront of developing community-based services for the homeless. With assistance from NIAAA, it created the CHARS Program, one of the first comprehensive service systems in the nation to address the needs of homeless individuals with alcohol and drug problems. Components of the system include an Alcohol Crisis Center, two Multi-purpose Drop-in Centers, Seven Residential Recovery Centers, a Transitional Housing Program, and Permanent Sober Housing.

One of the first such centers of its type in the nation, the 24 Hour Alcohol Crisis Center is designed to provide crisis and drop-in services for individuals currently experiencing alcohol-related problems, including those who are presently inebriated. Program elements include:

- *Inebriate Reception Center*: Located in downtown Oakland, the reception center provides a safe environment for public inebriates to escape from the street, rest, and sober up. Participants may include walk-in participants, and individuals brought in by police as a substitute for arrest for public intoxication. The center thus provides an alternative to the criminal justice system for public inebriates and offers a positive point of interaction with the alcohol recovery system. Referral to alcohol and drug programs and other needed services are made.
- *Refuge for people fleeing situations involving alcohol problems*: Housed with the Inebriate Reception Center but with a physically separate space, this component provides a place of

safety for individuals (predominantly women and their families) fleeing situations involving alcohol. Referrals to shelters, and emergency services will be offered. In addition, since many of those who come to this program have personal alcohol and drug problems, information about and referral to recovery services are also provided.

An initial request for proposals (RFP) for this component was issued in July, 1988. Only one organization chose to bid in response to this RFP; this single proposal was deemed by the review committee to be unacceptable. Feedback from alcohol services providers was solicited and incorporated into a revised RFP, which allowed greater subcontractor flexibility, and supplemented the contract amount with $60,000 in County funds. A number of proposals were received in response to this RFP, with the West Oakland Health Center being selected as the successful bidder in March 1989. In March, West Oakland Health Center obtained an excellent facility of 10,000 sq. ft. for the Crisis Center, located in downtown Oakland very close to a number of homeless shelters and meal sites, and within two blocks of Jefferson Park, where many homeless inebriates gather during the day.

Two Multipurpose Drop-in Centers offer homeless people with alcohol problems a primary point of entry for those seeking recovery or social services. Located in Oakland (in Northern Alameda County) and Newark (in Southern Alameda County) these Centers provide on-site alcohol and drug recovery services; shower and laundry facilities; one hot meal per day; information and referral to other alcohol and drug programs and social services; economic benefits counseling; telephone availability; transportation; and outreach to other agencies designed to facilitate the referral process.

The delivery of these services occurs in a warm, homelike, and safe atmosphere where homeless people can drop in to have a cup of coffee, visit, play cards, or just see a friendly welcoming face. Drop-in centers offer services based upon individual needs to those who desire them. When appropriate referrals are determined, appointments are made and referrals documented. Transportation is provided to detox and recovery services, if needed. Participants are encouraged to check in with the Center at least three times per week to participate in activities and to provide an opportunity for staff to follow-up on the participants' success in obtaining needed service. A mobile primary care van regularly visits the centers.

The drop-in centers were the first CHARS Program components in operation. Full program services began in July, 1988. In spite of a fire that totally destroyed the East Oakland Recovery Center facility in June, 1988, a new site was obtained and both have been providing services at a rate twice that envisioned in the original program design.

The East Oakland Recovery Center is currently providing a monthly average of 453 participant encounters to 135 (unduplicated) individuals in Oakland. Second Chance (in Newark) is currently providing 250 participant encounters to 34 individuals monthly. The Oakland Center operates 24 hours per day, while the Newark Center operates Monday through Friday, 8 am to 6 pm with crisis intervention and emergency transportation offered 24 hours per day through the Second Chance emergency shelter.

The Drop-in Centers are administered by Alameda County Department of Alcohol and Drug Programs (DADP) through the CHARS Program, but they are funded through Alameda County's Section 340 Health Care for the Homeless Program. In the process of negotiating the contract for these Centers, the Health Care for the Homeless Program and the CHARS Program have developed common automated data collection instruments and referral procedures. A common automated data system is currently under development that will provide the CHARS evaluation team with access health care and referral data on the 8,000 participants and 16,000 participant encounters in the Health Care for the Homeless System.

The County Residential Alcohol Recovery Program system has been redesigned to reduce barriers serving the homeless and to meet the increased demand for services generated by the CHARS Program. Upon renewal of each residential recovery center contract in July 1988, DADP included the stipulation that 25% of all recovery beds should be reserved for homeless participants, and that each residential recovery center should participate in CHARS data collection, outreach, and cross-training programs.

- Because twenty-five percent of the existing capacity of the County Residential Alcohol Recovery System has been reserved exclusively for the provision of immediate service to the homeless, the previous four to six week wait for program entry, which had been a major institutional barrier to the homeless, was reduced.
- A survey of residential recovery services in Alameda County conducted during the planning phase of the CHARS Program revealed that homeless individuals remained in residential recovery programs an average of 30% longer than necessary simply because the providers did not want to release them while they have no place to live. To meet the greatly increased demands upon the system to serve additional numbers of CHARS referrals, periods of residence at recovery centers have consequently been shortened where feasible, increasing the capacity of the Residential Recovery System by 25 to 50%. This shortened length of stay has been coupled with much more intensive assistance to participants leaving residential programs to assist them in finding housing, obtaining public benefits, and securing permanent employment.
- Interagency relationships between recovery centers and homeless service providers — including shelter, housing, health care and employment programs — have been established between staff of recovery centers and those of homeless programs. As a result, over 60% of the total participants in residential recovery are now homeless people. (See Table 1.)

Referrals are accepted directly from the drop-in centers, from homeless shelters and transitional programs, and from the Health Care for the Homeless Program. Providers are required to document provision of services to the homeless for each of the program beds committed to this program. Providers who refuse immediate service to a referral from a homeless agency must also document that either the referral was not appropriate for their services or that all of the reserved beds were full.

The Transitional Housing Component became operational June 30, 1988 with purchase of a 16 unit apartment complex, culminating several years of effort by SAVE, Inc. (an operator of a shelter for victims of domestic violence), Alameda County Housing and Community Development, and Alameda County DADP. This apartment complex supplements two existing transitional living programs for the homeless in Northern Alameda County. Participants include women who themselves are recovering and those who have been victims of another family member's alcohol problem, including victims of alcohol-related violence. This component provides families with up to eighteen months of residence, and offers on-site alcohol and drug recovery services, public benefits assistance, job search training, and assistance in securing vocational training. Participants are provided with vouchers to aid them in securing off-site childcare. They agree to maintain alcohol-free homes, and those who are themselves recovering from alcohol agree to participate regularly in community-based non-residential alcohol programs.

The Permanent Sober Housing component of CHARS assists participants to secure permanent housing by: helping to form stable households, and fill vacancies in existing households; aiding participants to locate affordable housing; accessing available loan and grant programs for tenant rental deposits; assisting community based organizations to assume financial and legal responsibilities for rentals in cases where participants simply cannot secure housing on their own behalf; and, proactively developing relationships with landlords, developers, and real estate agents to locate and secure moderately-priced rental housing.

Individuals are required to establish and maintain sober households as a condition for service under this program. They are assisted in obtaining non-residential recovery services, independent living services, employment training, and other relevant services by program staff who are also available for counseling and mediation should problems arise. By placing participants in commercial rental housing, rather than creating publicly-subsidized low-income housing, a number of disparate goals are achieved. First, many more placements can be achieved with the same funding. Secondly, living in commercial rental property gives participants the feeling that they are taking an additional step toward independence, and thirdly, renting commercial units at various locations assists them to re-enter mainstream society.

To implement this component an RFP to provide sober housing services was issued in July, 1988. A review committee meeting on September 14, 1988 recommended that SAVE, Inc. (also operators of the Transitional Housing Program) be awarded the contract. Board of Supervisors approval was obtained in October, and the contract was finalized in December, 1988.

Since January, 1989 the Permanent Sober Housing Program has been staffed by a full-time coordinator. The first several months of program operation were spent in outreach and resource development, location of landlords willing to cooperate with the program, and development of referral relationships with alcohol and homeless service providers. In March, the first month of direct participant services, thirteen families and individuals were placed in sober housing.

Finally, Alameda County has developed an unexcelled network of other support services for homeless and low-income people. The project draws fully upon these services to provide assistance to participants at all levels of the Comprehensive Homeless Alcohol Recovery Services Program. Among the major resources utilized are:

- *Health Care for the Homeless Project*: Housed in the Health Care Services Agency, the Health Care for the Homeless Project (HCHP) is both administratively and programmatically linked to the CHARS Program. Participants in alcohol recovery services not only have access to the primary and specialty medical care provided through HCHP, but are also offered case management and public benefits advocacy through HCHP. HCHP and CHARS are also developing a common participant data system to facilitate integrated service.

- *Non-Residential Alcohol Recovery Services*: Recovery from alcohol problems is not simply a matter of overcoming the addiction to alcohol. The development of alcohol problems is a process in which the individual severs ties with all aspects of life that do not involve drinking. Consequently, the recovering individual needs to recreate a life in which alcohol has no part.

    Each of the residential recovery programs involved in this project also offers non-residential recovery services, including counseling, recreation, and peer support activities. Non-residential recovery services are also available through 28 other programs in Alameda County. Although the process is somewhat different with each program, in each residential setting, the participant becomes acquainted with and involved in activities that he/she can continue on a non-residential basis. In this way, program participants are assisted to develop interests, friends, and recreations that support their independence from alcohol.

- *Additional Housing Services*: Even with the addition of the Transitional Housing Program, there is still a relative lack of transitional housing in Alameda County for program participants. This problem is being addressed in several ways:
  1. The Ninth Street Transitional House, a transitional living facility accepts referral of program participants in Northern Alameda County.
  2. The Sober Housing Program is designed to establish flexible housing arrangements tailored to the individual needs of program participants. Relatively large residences with peer support for a sober life style are being established as well as units occupied by single individuals or families. Alcohol counseling and support services for each of these houses is available through the non-residential services of the Department of Alcohol Programs.

- *Emergency Medical and Psychiatric Services*: For the Alcohol Crisis Center and for the Oakland Multipurpose Drop-In Center, these services are provided at (County-operated) Highland Hospital, West Oakland Health Center, and through the HCSA's Mobile Psychiatric Crisis Unit. Emergency Medical Services for the Newark Multipurpose Drop-In Center are provided through Washington Township Hospital in Newark, and Tri-Cities Health Center in Fremont.

In summary, CHARS reflects a significant effort to create a full continuum of community-based services for homeless people with alcohol and drug problems, and their families. The program does not simply treat participants' alcohol problems, only to release them back into a life of homelessness and desperation; nor does it provide only shelter without addressing the dependencies that bind individuals to a marginal lifestyle. Participant flow through the system is not based on a rigid set of program steps, but rather is flexible and tailored to the individual needs of each participant and his/her family. Rather than enforcing a specific model on the participant, this comprehensive approach to alcohol recovery stresses provision to each participant of the information and support necessary so that he/she can make his/her own life choices.

PROGRESS ACHIEVED

Aggregate Numbers — Table 1 compares initial participant service projections with actual services provided in the period July 1, 1988 through March 31, 1989 for the three programs that were fully implemented in this period: the Multipurpose Drop-In Centers, Residential Alcohol Recovery Programs, and Transitional Housing. Also provided are projections based upon these totals. It is clear from Table 1 that those CHARS Programs for which baseline data are available are performing at a capacity significantly above that originally projected.

Table 1. Comparison of Original Project Objectives, YTD Accomplishments, and Annualized Projects for Year Two

COMPONENT/ OBJECTIVE	Original Objective	Actual Performance 7/1/88 - 3/31/89	Annualized Projections
MULTIPURPOSE DROP-IN CENTERS			
Participants	900	1,385	1,600
Contacts	4,000	4,610	8,076
RECOVERY CENTERS			
Participants	174	446	600
Resident Days	20,000	21,206	31,809
TRANSITIONAL HOUSING			
Families	20	17	20
Units of Service	4,000	4,215	7,282

Intercomponent Referrals — It is clear that a very high proportion of the CHARS Program homeless participants are already accessing multiple project components. For example:

- 32.5% of Residential Recovery Center participants had utilized the drop-in centers prior to entering the residential program;
- 33.1% of CHARS Program participants in the period July to December, 1988 had also utilized non alcohol-related services provided by the Health Care for the Homeless Program. Of these, 24.7% had received primary care services, and 23.6% had utilized case management services.

Considering the restricted time frame covered by these analyses, the numbers show a significant utilization by participants of multiple service components within the CHARS Program and between the CHARS Program and associated components of the Health Care for the Homeless System.

System Building and Community Linkages — In the social-community model of alcohol recovery services upon which the CHARS Program is based, success of program services is dependent not so much on a formal structure of procedures and "interventions" as upon the provision of an array of services from which recovering individuals may develop alternate paths to recovery specific to their particular needs and circumstances, and upon the nurturance of a community of attitudes and relationships which promote constructive personal choices by recovering individuals.

The success of this service delivery model depends not so much on formal referral mechanisms, interagency agreements, service protocols, etc. as upon the creation of an information-rich environment on the level of individual programs and service providers and upon the creation of a culture of cooperation and commitment to the recovery process among participants, providers, and program administrators. Nevertheless, the county has formal contracts with each service provider who is a part of the CHARS program. Each contract delineates specific, measurable performance objectives. There is also a comprehensive specific written protocol for oversight of these contracts.

One of the major accomplishments of the CHARS Program in its first year of operation has been catalyzing the growing cooperation and mutual understanding of homeless service programs and alcohol recovery services. This has been accomplished through a vigorous program of outreach activities and staff training undertaken by CHARS administration and by each of the components of the CHARS Program. Within the period between July 1988 and January 1989, the CHARS Program participated in nearly 200 outreach activities and information sharing sessions encompassing:

- 22 alcohol- and drug-services providers;
- 18 homeless shelters;
- 21 other organizations providing homeless services;
- 13 community-based primary care programs;
- numerous other community groups, landlord and business associations, and police departments.

In addition, CHARS has become an active member of the Emergency Services Network, a coalition of 104 service providers in Alameda County. DADP holds monthly meetings of all CHARS Providers which combine presentations on topics of general interest with specific discussions of program coordination, cooperation, and integration.

CHARS EVALUATION

The program evaluation does not confine itself to rote quantification of services rendered, but is attempting to describe and explain the processes and problems of program implementation, and to document the paths to recovery or failure experienced by program participants. Major research issues addressed by the CHARS evaluation include:

Characteristics of the Target Population — The project is attempting to specify — at a minimum — demographics and social characteristics of the target population, and to quantify the extent to which the demographic and social characteristics of homeless people with alcohol and drug problems differ from that of the general homeless population in Alameda County.

Patterns of Service Utilization—From the general target population, which subgroups utilize particular program components? What factors lead these subgroups to seek services? What factors in the lives of individuals lead them to seek recovery services, and what factors lead them to succeed in recovery services? What economic, institutional, social, and/or psychological barriers restrict access to services among the homeless populations?

Actual Processes of Service Delivery—How were services actually delivered? How did this differ from the original program design? What factors shaped the actual implementation, and what factors aided or impeded the achievement of program goals?

Referral Patterns and Referral Utilization—What were the patterns of external referrals? What factors lead some agencies or types of agencies to make substantial numbers of referrals, and others to make few referrals? What were the factors which determined the services to which particular individuals would be referred? How can the referral process be optimized? What percentages of referrals were actually acted on by the individual referred? What factors lead individuals to follow-up or to not follow-up on program referrals?

Service Delivery—What were the actual quantity of services delivered? Which services were effective in assisting participants, and which were not effective? What were the reasons for success or failure? To what extent did outreach efforts, provider training, institutional adjustments, and other factors affect the increase/decrease in program utilization by homeless people over the period of the project?

The evaluation design combines computer-based participant tracking and quantification of service activities with structured interviews of key actors in the system including service providers, program administrators, staff of emergency shelters, meal sites, police departments, other potential referral sources, and program participants.

Participant Tracking—At the point of entry into each program component and upon transfer from one component to another, an entry form is completed for each participant. Considerable sensitivity to the needs and time demands of program staff and to the dignity of individual respondents has been shown in the development of data collection instruments. Earlier versions were reviewed by

CHARS providers and administrators and their suggestions incorporated. The form contains the following key variables: birthdate, sex, ethnicity, family status, number of children under 18, number of children residing with parent, ages of children residing with parent, type of current residence, how long homeless, previous homelessness, employment status, monthly income, veteran status, primary language spoken, and referral source.

In addition to the entry form, residential recovery centers complete exit information on each participant leaving the program. This includes: participant name, exit date, reason for departure, employment status at exit, and housing status at exit.

Each of the variables used in the entry and exit forms is consistent with those employed by the Emergency Services Network (ESN) in its annual study of the general homeless population. The CHARS Program also utilizes ESN raw survey data to determine what proportion of the overall homeless population access its services, and to assess demographic similarities and differences between the target population and the general homeless population.

In addition to participant entry and referral forms which are provided by all program components, a number of supplemental data forms are maintained by the individual program components, as appropriate for the type of service offered. Moreover, the CHARS Program, because it can link its own project data with the Health Care for the Homeless Project data, will be able to develop a health status profile of CHARS participants and to compare that profile to the health status of the general homeless population of Alameda County.

Qualitative Observations — In addition to the data collection described above, the Program evaluators are collecting qualitative information through "structured field work," i.e., participant observation, and intensive interviewing. This effort will provide a community case history of the implementation and long-term viability of CHARS.

In conclusion, the CHARS program seeks to facilitate positive lifestyle changes at the individual level by providing opportunities and environments that facilitate recovery from alcohol problems. Systems level changes are of critical importance to the success of the program. Ongoing program development will continue to focus on increasing system-wide awareness of the nature and scope of alcohol problems among homeless people as well as strategies to improve access to and utilization of services available.

BIBLIOGRAPHY

Garrett, Gerald R. 1989 "Once over lightly: An historical overview of research on alcohol problems and homelessness." Paper for the conference on Homelessness, Alcohol, and Other Drugs held in San Diego, CA.

Gelberg, Lillian, Lawrence S. Linn and Barbara D. Leake 1988 "Mental health, alcohol and drug use, and criminal history among homeless adults." *American Journal of Psychiatry* 145:191-196.

Hawkins, J. David, Denise M. Lishner, Jeffrey Jenson, and Richard F. Catalano 1986 "Delinquents and drugs: What the evidence suggests about prevention and treatment programming." Paper prepared for NIDA Technical Review Meeting on Special Youth Populations.

Kaufman, Nancy 1989 "Access to housing for homeless substance abusers." Paper for the conference on Homelessness, Alcohol, and Other Drugs held in San Diego, CA.

Moskowitz, Joel M. 1984 "The primary prevention of alcohol problems: A critical review of the research literature." *Primary Prevention*

National Institute on Drug Abuse 1983 *Handbook for Prevention Evaluation: Prevention Evaluation Guidelines*

Piliavin, Irving 1989 "Stayers and leavers among the homeless: Some recent findings." Paper for the conference on Homelessness, Alcohol, and Other Drugs held in San Diego, CA.

Stark, Louisa 1987 "A century of alcohol and homelessness: demographics and stereotypes." *Alcohol Health and Research World* 2(3): 8-13.

U.S. Dept. of Education 1987 Report to Congress and the White House on the Nature and Effectiveness of Federal, State, and Local Drug Prevention Education Programs.

Wright, James D. and Eleanor Weber 1988 "Determinants of benefit-program participation among the urban homeless." *Evaluation Review* 12(4):376-395.

Family Treatment for Homeless Alcohol/Drug-Addicted Women and Their Preschool Children

Marilee Comfort, MPH, PhD
Thomas E. Shipley, Jr., PhD
Kathleen White, MS
Ellen M. Griffith, MHA
Irving W. Shandler, MA, MSW

Substance abuse treatment programs are facing a major change in client profiles. Cocaine, or cocaine combined with alcohol, is rapidly joining the ranks of alcohol and heroin as a primary drug of abuse. By the last quarter of 1987, cocaine had surpassed heroin and alcohol as the drug of choice for all clients in Philadelphia's public treatment programs. Cocaine admissions to these programs have more than doubled annually since 1984, from 439 to almost 7,657 in 1988 (Hoerlin, 1989). Women, in particular, are seeking treatment for cocaine addiction in increasing numbers. Between 1980 and 1988, the number of female admissions to substance abuse programs in Philadelphia increased from 22 to 2505 (Wiegand, 1988). Data from one of these programs, the Diagnostic and Rehabilitation Center of Philadelphia (DRC), show cocaine as the primary drug of abuse for 87% of the female clients and for 76% of the male clients (Diagnostic and Rehabilitation Center, 1989).

Marilee Comfort, Kathleen White, Ellen M. Griffith and Irving W. Shandler are affiliated with the Diagnostic and Rehabilitation Center, 229 Arch Street, Philadelphia, PA 19106. Thomas E. Shipley, Jr. is on the faculty of the Department of Psychology, Temple University, Weiss Hall, Philadelphia, PA 19122.

The authors wish to give special thanks to the DRC Staff and Clients who graciously participated in the Demonstration Project Pilot Study.

The increased prevalence of cocaine use by women, particularly those of childbearing age, triggers special concern for pregnant women, mothers and children. The National Association for Perinatal Addiction Research and Education estimates 10%, or 375,000 newborns each year are exposed to illicit drugs before birth (State of NJ, 1989). Cocaine use during pregnancy is being reported with increasing frequency. In a 1987 survey conducted by the National Cocaine Hotline, 20% of the female callers reported cocaine use during pregnancy. In Boston, a prospective study of cocaine use during pregnancy found that 17 percent of women enrolled in prenatal care had used cocaine at least once during pregnancy (Frank et al., 1988). A recent medical chart review of 1000 mothers and newborns from eight Philadelphia hospitals revealed that 16.3% of mothers had used cocaine (Philadelphia Perinatal Society, 1989). This figure is considered a conservative estimate due to maternal underreporting which is typical when drug use is documented by verbal report alone (Hingson et al., 1986).

Added to the abuse of cocaine is the continued problem of alcohol abuse. A third of the 10 to 18 million alcoholics in the United States in 1984 were women. Given the general acceptance of drinking in American society and the covert style of drinking that women tend to adopt, identification of female alcoholics is difficult, but again, especially critical when a women is pregnant. Two to thirteen percent of pregnant women have been identified as heavy drinkers. Among heavy drinkers, figures ranging from 1 to 43 percent of pregnant women, have been associated with Fetal Alcohol Syndrome in the medical literature. Of the 40 percent of pregnant women who are moderate drinkers, 11 to 19 percent deliver babies with abnormalities similar to FAS (Mullins & Gazaway, 1985). The wide variability in prevalence translates into uncertainty in the minds of pregnant women, who may then discount warnings about alcohol consumption during pregnancy and subsequent breastfeeding.

Current research on the perinatal effects of cocaine suggests that even if the cocaine problem were solved today, the drug's adverse impact would be felt by society for another generation. Babies born to cocaine users show increased incidence of a number of health problems, most notably decreased gestational age, low birth weight, and small head circumference. Furthermore, neonatal characteristics associated with cocaine use such as irritability, tremulousness, abnormal sleep patterns, and muted alertness can interfere with early family relations (Finnegan et al., 1989). Further research is necessary to clarify the precursors to these problems in development and family functioning. Meanwhile, the multifaceted impact of a developmentally disabled child is felt by the child, the parent, the family and society for a life-time.

Clearly, women's increased use of cocaine and alcohol and their potential effects on children and families indicate a pressing need for timely intervention with substance-abusing women. In 1987, just over a quarter of the individuals admitted to Philadelphia treatment programs were women, although they represented nearly half of the cocaine-related emergency room visits. That discrepancy suggests that many more women would be in treatment if spaces were available and if programs acknowledged women's particular issues when seeking help.

Women, Children and Substance Abuse Among the Homeless

Substance abuse is becoming increasingly apparent in homeless populations. There is a growing recognition among advocates, public officials and service providers that an exceedingly high percentage of the homeless, estimates ranging from 10 to 40 percent, abuse alcohol or drugs (Committee on Health Care, 1988). While substance abuse afflicts all classes and races, the crack epidemic has especially pervaded economically disadvantaged, non-white urban neighborhoods. The impact of drug and alcohol abuse is manifested in numerous areas of society, of which homelessness and child morbidity/mortality are two prime examples. Family finances are dissipated by cocaine or alcohol. Domestic violence and child abuse are frequent correlates of substance abuse. Mothers may forget they are mothers when addicted to crack. Anecdotal reports vividly describe how families are disrupted, parenting responsibilities are easily ignored and children are neglected when mothers are addicted to cocaine (Gross, 1989; Howard et al., 1989; Ehrlich & Finnegan, 1987; Weigand, 1989).

It is no coincidence that as cocaine addiction increases among women, the number of women among the homeless population is on the rise. The homeless population used to consist primarily of alcoholic men. Today, the Committee on Health Care for Homeless People of the Institute of Medicine (1988) reports that families with children are the most quickly escalating subgroup among the homeless in the United States today. Families, usually women with two or three children, make up an estimated 28 percent of the homeless population nationwide (Sullivan & Damrosch, 1987). The dramatic impact of homelessness and cocaine on women and children presents a new challenge for the Diagnostic and Rehabilitation Center of Philadelphia which has 26 years of experience in drug and alcohol treatment.

THE DIAGNOSTIC AND REHABILITATION CENTER OF PHILADELPHIA

Purpose and Philosophy

The central mission of the DRC is to provide services for substance abuse recovery, primarily to those who are indigent and eligible for public welfare — poor, homeless and/or chronically ill persons. Through a comprehensive array of services, the DRC seeks to break the cycle of drug and welfare dependency. Initially, services concentrate on meeting the physical needs of food, clothing, and medical care. Therapy then focuses on gaining and maintaining sobriety. Concurrently, help is given to solve the multitude of practical and emotional problems which have precipitated or have been aggravated by addiction.

In general, many substance abusers present similar problems including: poor self-esteem, lack of internal motivation and direction, a disorganized family that may be abusive and addictive, difficulty finding and sustaining employment, social or emotional problems. The DRC believes that these people can be motivated to change and to remain sober or drug free and learn the skills and supports necessary to achieve independence and stability. Through access to a wide range of resources, enough time for the client to gain the strength to move toward sobriety and realistic goals for both the client and the agency, the DRC staff believes that successful recovery is possible.

Program Overview

The DRC was established in 1963 as a private, not-for-profit agency, in conjunction with Temple University, the Greater Philadelphia Movement, and the City of Philadelphia. Since its beginning, the DRC has provided comprehensive services for substance abusers. At first, the agency's primary concern was with the "skid row" population. Over the years the DRC has built a reputation as a free-standing substance abuse agency which offers services to the homeless and those in lower socioeconomic strata of society.

The DRC provides a variety of services including medically-supervised residential detoxification, diagnostic and emergency medical services, partial hospitalization programs, bridge housing, and shelter for homeless men. The DRC also offers comprehensive outpatient treatment for alcohol or drug addiction, with drop-in childcare while parents attend treatment sessions at the DRC.

The Women's Program at the DRC is especially tailored to women's needs in the areas of substance abuse, interpersonal relations, job-training, and housing. Bridge housing is offered to women in need of a supervised alcohol/drug-free environment while preparing for independent living and entry into the job market. After graduation from outpatient treatment, women are encouraged to maintain contact with the client-run Aftercare program coordinated by the DRC staff (see Shandler & Shipley, 1987 for more detailed information about the DRC). To attempt to meet the new challenges of cocaine and homelessness, the DRC has opened a residential family treatment program for homeless polydrug-addicted women with preschool children.

DRC Demonstration Project Overview

The DRC Demonstration Project is funded by the National Institute for Alcohol Abuse and Alcoholism (NIAAA) to examine the efficacy of transitional family housing and treatment on homeless, alcohol/drug-addicted women and their preschool children. One hundred and twenty women and their children under six years of age will be studied prospectively as they proceed through the treatment process. The project provides transitional housing for the family in conjunction with outpatient counseling and referral services for the mothers.

The eligibility criteria for admission to the DRC Demonstration Project are as follows:

— Women 18 years of age or older
— Pregnant women or mothers with pre-school children in their care
— Alcohol or drug problems
— Homeless or at imminent risk of becoming homeless
— Ambulatory and able to physically care for themselves and their children
— No recent evidence of violent or psychotic behavior.

Referrals are accepted from the DRC's Detoxification and Outpatient programs, the Philadelphia shelter system, local medical centers and from the Department of Human Services. The families are randomly assigned to the residential or non-residential programs. After the mother is detoxified, the family is welcomed into the residence and oriented to the house guidelines. Each family is assigned sleeping accommodations designed to provide a sense of privacy and personal space.

Residential Program

Training in life skills is incorporated into the residential program in such basic areas as nutrition, shopping, food preparation, parenting and maintenance of the environment. While in the residence, each client is expected to invest time and energy into the operation of the facility. It is not the intention of this project to take responsibility for the care of women and their children. Instead, each client learns to be responsible for herself and for her children by cleaning her own area, and laundering her family's clothing. Meals are prepared and common living areas are maintained by all of the women on a rotating basis. The purchase and preparation of food is overseen by the staff with emphasis on the nutritional and economic needs of the families in residence. This participatory approach is designed to teach the women how to manage their families' daily needs. Daily meetings are held among the women and the residential staff in order to assign chores and process the issues of living together. In this manner these issues do not occupy therapeutic time and problem solving is implemented immediately and directly with the persons involved.

All clients engage in cooperative babysitting, closely supervised by the the Residential Staff. When clients are scheduled for therapy at the DRC outpatient treatment facility, they take their children with them to the DRC Child Care Services. Those women not scheduled for outpatient appointments on a particular day help manage the children at the residence.

Within the residence, alternative strategies for child care and management are explored individually and parenting skills training is provided for staff and clients in group sessions. With the assistance of parenting consultants, incidental family problems are processed by the families and staff, thus applying skills training to daily experiences in the residence. Families are referred to outside agencies for health, financial, legal, social and child development services, as necessary. Any health or developmental problems identified by program evaluation assessments or staff observations are discussed at case consultations to determine whether there is a need for referral to community services. The women in the residence are assisted by a Resource Development Specialist in utilizing community services.

Although the length of stay in the residence will vary across families, six months is the anticipated average. Exit dates will be carefully planned by means of consultation between the DRC's Residential Staff and Outpatient Treatment Staff. The pace through the program will be determined by the progress of the individual family in the residential and therapeutic components of the program.

Therapeutic Treatment for Addiction

In addition to the residential program for families, the women receive therapeutic treatment for addiction. The DRC brings six years of experience in treatment of addicted women to this Demonstration Project. Therapy proceeds in four phases according to the client's individual needs throughout the treatment process. Phase One forms the foundation for recovery which includes: (1) education regarding addiction and its power; (2) introduction to group processing; (3) financial stabilization; (4) access to medical care; and (5) safe, sober housing when possible.

In Phase Two, therapy becomes more intense and the counselor attempts to help the client focus on feelings and personal responsibility, while building support systems within and outside of the DRC. In this phase, an attempt is made to help clients relate to other women, to gain an understanding of themselves and to decrease their isolation.

Phase Three involves intensive group therapy, usually focused on unresolved issues such as sexual abuse, physical abuse, dysfunctions experienced by adult children of alcoholics and low self-esteem.

Phase-out occurs in the fourth and final phase. To enter Phase Four the client must have developed outside support systems. In this phase, relapse prevention is emphasized and the concerns of separation between counselor and client are resolved. After treatment is completed, Aftercare involves referral for vocational training, academic training, or on-going counseling in specific areas such as parent-child relations.

Project Evaluation

The project evaluation is designed to describe and compare the characteristics and outcomes of two groups of women with preschool children over a 12-month period: (1) 60 families in the residential program (R) who receive supervised transitional housing and outpatient services; and (2) 60 families in the non-residential program (NR) who receive only outpatient services. The evaluation study will compare the personal and family outcomes of mothers in the R and NR groups as a function of individual characteristics such as alcohol/drug use patterns, housing history, perceived stress and support, and family relations. In addition, the children's developmental progress will be monitored. Process outcomes will include descriptions of the DRC Residential and Outpatient services, service utilization patterns and community linkages. (A detailed description of the Evaluation Plan is available from the authors.)

Case Management and Ancillary Services

Previous experience gained from the DRC's other residential programs suggests that intensive case management is essential to effectively address the needs of addicted women and their families. Community linkages have been developed to access direct services for mothers and children ranging from health care and education to legal, financial and child welfare services. Most women at the DRC have had negative experiences with community agencies and require a case manager to accompany them initially to appointments to teach them how to access and use the resources in the community.

Currently, assistance with securing safe, drug-free, affordable housing is the most difficult community service to access. The few public and private agencies that handle housing requests are overloaded with requests and have limited resources. As an alternative to single-family living, the DRC encourages clients to share housing, thereby pooling their resources and offering mutual support for maintaining drug-free lifestyles.

To coordinate the numerous linkages developed in the community during the DRC's long history of treating substance-abusing individuals, the DRC Demonstration Project instigated an Advisory Council for the Women's Program. The members were selected from the medical, legal, financial, social service and education professions in order to facilitate communication between the DRC and the Philadelphia community.

In summary, the overall aim of the DRC Demonstration Project is to assist women in learning basic personal and family living skills which can be carried with them into the community. They also will be assisted in furthering their education and entering vocational training or the job market. The intent of the project is to go beyond simply sheltering families by helping them to develop the tools necessary for constructive independent lives. The project aims to encourage each woman to understand her addiction, develop a strong support system, and establish stable emotional relationships with her children while living in a supportive group setting. The next step is to foster separation from the program and independent living in the community. Accomplishment of these aims requires delivery of integrated counseling, residential, and evaluation services in which staff efforts are coordinated by a team approach.

DRC PILOT STUDY

The Demonstration Project Research Staff conducted a Pilot Study designed to describe the characteristics, attitudes and treatment of a sample of DRC women comparable to the clients proposed for the Demonstration Project. Women were recruited from three treatment programs within the DRC in order to compare clients receiving different types of services—detoxification, outpatient, and residential services. At the DRC the Detoxification program serves as an entry program which helps alleviate immediate physical and emotional needs and introduces the clients to the longer-term treatment programs. The Outpatient Program and the Next Step residential program provide long-term treatment for those clients who have made a commitment to abstain from alcohol or drugs for several weeks or more.

The Pilot Study allowed the Research Staff a glimpse of the people, policies, procedures and channels of communication within the DRC, as well as linkages with outside agencies, in preparation for the subsequent evaluation study. This brief report of results highlights profiles of the alcohol and drug use history, affective reactions, family history and the support system of a sample of DRC female clients.

Method

Data were collected between November, 1988 and February, 1989 from 66 homeless polydrug-addicted women distributed among three DRC treatment programs as follows: (1) Detoxification Unit (DTX) (N = 38), (2) Outpatient Program (OP) (N = 13), (3) Next Step, a residential program (NS) (N = 15). A client was interviewed if she was residing in an unstable living situation, had children and was willing to participate in two interview sessions with the Research Staff.

Semi-structured interviews were developed to complement the overview information gathered with the Addiction Severity Index (McLellan et al., 1985). The interviews included open- and closed-ended questions regarding demographics, housing history, alcohol/ drug use patterns and attitudes, and history of and attitudes toward treatment. Other items examined the family history, social support, and personal and family needs and goals.

This report presents findings from the Addiction Severity Index (ASI) (N = 66) and the Housing/Family/Treatment Interview (HFT) (N = 56). The smaller number of respondents for the HFT reflects second appointments missed by clients. Comparisons of interest will be made among clients in the three treatment programs.

RESULTS

Demographics

Ninety-two percent of the 66 clients in the pilot study are black. The ages range from late teens to early forties, averaging 28 (DTX), 30 (OP) and 28 (NS) years of age. The groups do not show wide discrepancies in educational attainment. The average grade completed in school (ranging from 8 years to a Master's degree) was approximately 11th grade; the OP group averaged slightly lower, and the Detoxification group averaged slightly higher educational attainment. The majority of OP (85%) and NS (73%) clients, and approximately half of the DTX clients (55%) receive public assistance funds.

Approximately three-fourths of the entire sample has never been married. Only three of the clients are currently married. The women have an average of 2 to 3 children, almost half of whom (46%) are less than 6 years old and the majority of whom (83%) are less than 13 years old. Forty-six percent of the women have given up custody of a child (primarily to relatives) at some time in their lives.

During the past five years, the number of times clients changed residences ranged from 0 to 20 times; one to six moves being most typical. The women in NS average more than twice the moves cited by OP clients and a slightly higher average than the DTX clients.

Alcohol and Drug Use

A wide variety of drugs have been used with regularity over the lifetime by this sample. The drugs used most heavily were alcohol, marijuana, and cocaine. Ninety-two percent of the entire sample reported heavy use of cocaine. The average number of years of heavy use for DTX clients is twice that of the OP clients, whereas heavy use of alcohol is twice as prevalent in the OP group as in the DTX group.

The history of heavy alcohol and drug use is substantially different between the relatively stable, long-term treatment clients (OP and NS) and the newer DTX clients. The former show a much longer history of heavy use of alcohol and marijuana with a relatively shorter involvement with cocaine. Their reports of prior treatment for alcohol and drugs reinforce that picture, showing a particularly striking difference in prior treatment for alcohol abuse. Fewer DTX clients (16%) than OP (69%) or NS (47%) clients reported prior treatment for alcohol problems.

In addition to alcohol/drug use and treatment, another index of how deeply involved the women are in the drug culture is the amount of money spent on drugs in the prior month. The DTX group's reports ranged from $100 to $7000, with most clients reporting $100-$900 spent in a month. The amount of money spent on drugs correlates highly with the amount of illegal money received for those who reported such income ($r = +.87$, $P < .01$).

Affective Reactions

The prevalence of negative affect associated with alcohol and drug addiction is reflected in reports of depression, anxiety, hallucinations or suicidal thoughts during the prior month from 77% of OP, 87% of NS and 97% DTX clients. Lifetime reports of these dysphoric symptoms, suggest that unpleasant mood tends to be salient for all of the clients, but especially for the Detoxification clients of whom 87% recalled symptoms.

Family History

Most of the clients were raised by their biological mothers and fathers (50%) or by biological mothers alone (21%). The remaining women were raised by biological mothers and stepfathers, other relatives, or a combination of two of the above. The women in each program recalled substantial numbers of alcohol or drug problems within their families, with the highest percentages noted by OP clients (55% mothers, 82% fathers). Problems were perceived more so for fathers or other family members than for mothers.

Sixty-four percent of the total sample recalled experiencing abuse by someone during childhood in the forms of verbal, physical and/ or sexual abuse. Abuse attributed to mother, father and others (mostly family members) is highest in the NS group (38%, 38%, 70%). Twenty-one to 31% of DTX and OP clients reported abuse from the three sources above; except the OP group, for whom 44% of clients reported paternal abuse.

Social Support

Despite family histories of alcohol or drug problems and abuse, the clients perceived a great deal of support from their families. The majority of women reported strong family support for emotional needs. Many of the supportive persons named were the client's mother or other family members, such as siblings or children. DTX and NS clients claimed friends as a much stronger source of support than did OP clients. Professionals and organized groups were cited as supportive most often by OP and NS clients, those in long-term treatment programs.

DISCUSSION

The Pilot Study offers insights into the lives of young minority urban mothers who are actively struggling with intergenerational cycles of substance abuse, child abuse, disorganized families and few environmental resources. This represents a snapshot of the participants in the DRC Demonstration Project, that is, homeless poly-drug-addicted mothers in treatment for alcohol and drug problems. On the average, this sample is composed of unmarried black women in their late twenties with varying histories of alcohol and drug use who have discovered cocaine relatively recently. With the sudden escalation in cocaine abuse, there is a tendency to forget that other problem substances such as alcohol, heroin, marijuana and tobacco, have not disappeared. Almost all of the women have had at least one prior treatment for alcohol or drugs. Most of the clients report histories of adverse affective symptoms and, like other studies of drug-abusing women, many personal and family adjustment problems (Glenn & Parsons, 1989; Lief, 1985; Regan, Ehrlich & Finnegan, 1987).

Clinical observations by the Women's Treatment Staff characterize recent cocaine-addicted clients as less stable in their living situations, more difficult to engage in treatment, and prone to drop out of treatment more quickly and more frequently than the traditional alcoholic. Many of the women appear to lack a general sense of appropriate behavior, resort easily to physical violence and are verbally abusive. In seeking "in-patient" treatment they seem to be seeking a safe place to live as much as they are seeking treatment for addiction. In spite of their aggressiveness and lack of control, they are frightened in the current shelter system. Generally, these mothers are unsure of how to deal with their children and want to be removed from the addictive and abusive environments that have contributed to their own addiction and to the potential abuse and addiction of their children. The impact of the needs of these women and families can be seen in the growing waiting lists for the DRC women's Detoxification Unit, Outpatient Services and Next Step Program.

The Pilot Study findings suggest that the three women's treatment programs within the DRC (DTX, OP and NS) are dealing with clients of significantly different profiles which may require varied approaches to treatment. For example, the alcohol and drug use histories of the groups differ markedly. In general, the members of the OP and NS groups tend to report greater prior involvement and treatment for alcohol than the DTX group. Of course, one obvious difference between the DTX group and the other two groups is stability in treatment. The OP and NS groups, by definition of the services, have demonstrated greater responsibility in treatment by maintaining sobriety for an extended period and ongoing commitments with counselors, support groups and community agencies. In contrast, only 22% of the DTX clients in the Pilot Study remained in the OP program a month after the study was conducted.

There are at least two possible explanations for the differences in histories of alcohol and drug use and treatment of the groups. The first reason, denial, suggests that the DTX clients have as severe a problem with alcohol as the members of the other groups, but that they deny the severity of the problems with drugs other than cocaine. On the other hand, through treatment, the members of the long-term groups (OP and NS) have come to recognize the severity of their problems with several drugs.

A second explanation suggests that those with longer histories with several drugs have cycled through abuse and treatment to the point that they are desperate to find a non-drug solution to their problems. That is to say, they have "hit bottom." Hence, they are more apt to enter a long-term treatment program after detoxification and to remain longer in treatment.

In the Pilot Study, the OP and NS groups reported greater involvement with several drugs, a greater number of prior treatments, as well as longer participation in the present treatment episode than the DTX group. Regardless of the explanation for the differences in history, DTX clients require sensitive and timely support for the decision to continue into long-term treatment. Careful coordination of referrals between programs and substantial incentives to continue are clearly necessary to ensure that DTX clients enter and maintain stability in long-term treatment.

Practitioners and researchers in the treatment community are only beginning to appreciate the magnitude of the complex interactions involved in the addiction and recovery processes. It is clear from the Pilot Study findings and other reports that ours is now a polydrug-abusing society. Drug use is certainly influenced strongly by socio-economic conditions, personal characteristics and family patterns (Glenn & Parsons, 1989; Regan, Ehrlich & Finnegan, 1987; Weston et al., 1989).

Among the multitude of problems experienced by homeless alcohol/drug-addicted women, the DRC women identified two primary family concerns: (1) having a safe place to live independently with their children and (2) developing close relationships with their children. These are not surprising, given the risks to early parent-child relations presented in these families. These concerns are confirmed by other studies of homeless or drug-addicted mothers (Bassuk, 1986; Bauman & Dougherty, 1983; Boxill, 1989; Fiks, Johnson & Rosen, 1985). Boxill and Beatty (1987) describe mothers in Atlanta shelters who "are forced by circumstance to define themselves and build their mother/child relationships in an open and public, personal place" (p. 136). Beginning with a disorganized lifestyle, the addicted mother frequently has difficulty meeting the needs of herself and her children in what typically is a stressful environment with few personal, social or financial resources (Lief, 1985).

It follows logically that a major theme expressed by DRC women when listing treatment needs was social support. This confirms other recent studies of homeless and drug-addicted women (Bassuk & Rosenberg, 1988; Regan, Ehrlich & Finnegan, 1987). Support from multiple sources appears to be valuable to DRC women in coping with the pressures of their lives. However, family members were mentioned as supports most frequently by all three groups, despite the high incidence of family alcohol/drug problems and abusive relationships that could limit the responsiveness of family members. Given the striking burden of unanticipated grandchild care described by San Francisco mothers of cocaine-addicted women (Gross, 1989), one wonders whether the consistent reports of family support may sometimes be more idealized than real. These addicted mothers may be drawing too heavily on their families for daily support. During recovery, the usual sources of parenting support, that is family or friends, may not be able to provide the intense specialized guidance needed by cocaine-addicted parents to reorganize their lives and interactions with their children.

The threat presented by cocaine, or its more highly addictive derivative, crack, looms large in many urban families. Cocaine has been described as one of the most reinforcing, if not the most reinforcing and addicting drug that has ever been studied in modern medicine (State of NJ, 1989). Its impact is being felt throughout the health and social service systems (French, 1989; Hoerlin, 1989).

There is an urgent need for family-oriented treatment approaches which address cocaine addiction, homelessness, as well as family relationships and support issues. This point is corroborated loudly and clearly by national reviews of programs for high risk, low resource families (Healthy Mothers, Healthy Babies, 1986; Kagan, Powello, Weissbourd & Zigler, 1987; Schorr, 1988). Successful treatment programs offer comprehensive, high-intensity services and establish relationships with families built on mutual respect and trust (Howard et al., 1989). It is critical that these programs be tailored to the individual needs of families with diverse histories and problems.

Based on prior experience within the DRC and the results of the Pilot Study, the DRC Demonstration Project will place high priority on the development of procedures and incentives which promote treatment stability for homeless, addicted women with children. We propose that providing these families with a transitional residence while the mothers are involved in treatment for addiction will offer a fundamental incentive and much of the support necessary to establish personal and family stability without drugs and alcohol.

REFERENCES

Bauman, P.S., & Dougherty, F.E. (1983). Drug addicted mothers' parenting and their children's development. *International Journal of the Addictions*, *18*, 291-302.

Bassuk, E.L. (1986). Homeless families: Single mothers and their children in Boston shelters. In Bassuk, E. (Ed.), *Mental Health Needs of Homeless Persons*, No. 30 in the series "New Directions for Mental Health Services" San Francisco; Jossey-Bass, Inc.

Bassuk, E.L., & Rosenberg, L. (1988). Why does family homelessness occur? A case-control study. *American Journal of Public Health*, *78* (7), 783-788.

Boxill, N.A., & Beaty, A.L. (1987). An exploration of mother/child interaction among homeless women and their children using a public night shelter in Atlanta, Georgia. In *The crisis in homelessness: Effects on children and families*. Hearing before the Select Committee on Children, Youth, and Families, House of Representatives, One Hundredth Congress, Pub. No. 72-237. Washington, D.C.: U.S. Government Printing Office.

Boxill, N.A., & Board of Commissioners, Fulton County, Georgia (1989). Forming human connections in shelters for homeless women and children. *Zero to Three*, *9*, pp. 19-21.

Committee on Health Care, Institute of Medicine (1988). *Homelessness, health, and human needs*. Washington, D.C.: National Academy Press.

Diagnostic and Rehabilitation Center of Philadelphia (1989). *Third Quarter Statistical Report*. Philadelphia, Pa.

Fiks, K.B., Johnson, H.L., & Rosen, T.S. (1985) Methadone-maintained mothers: 3-year follow-up of parental functioning. *International Journal of Addictions, 20*, 651-660.

Finnegan, L.P., Mellott, J.M., Ryan, L.M., & Wapner, R.J. (1989, in press). Perinatal exposure to cocaine: Human studies. In J.M. Lakoski, M.P. Galloway and F.J. White (eds.) *Cocaine: Pharmacology, Physiology and Clinical Strategies.*

Frank, D.A., Zuckerman, B.S., Amaro, H., Akboagye, K., Bauchner, H., Cabral, H., Fried, L., Hingson, R., Kayne, H., Levenson, S.M., Parker, S., Reece, H., & Vinci, R. (1988, December). Cocaine use during pregnancy: Prevalence and Correlates. *Pediatrics, 32* (6), 888-895.

French, H.W. (May 10, 1989). Crack filling New York hospitals with frustration, fear and crime. *New York Times*, A1 & B5.

Glenn, S.W., & Parsons, O.A.l (1989). Alcohol abuse and familial alcoholism: Psychosocial correlates in men and women. *Journal of Studies on Alcohol, 50,* 116-127.

Gross, J. (April 8, 1989). Grandmothers bear a burden sired by drugs. *New York Times*, pp. 1, 26.

Healthy Mothers, Healthy Babies. (1986). *A compendium for serving low-income women*, DHHS Publication No. (PHS) 86-50209, Washington, D.C. Superintendent of Documents, U.S. Government Printing Office.

Hingson, R., Zuckerman, B., Amaro, H., Frank, D., Kayne, H., Sorenson, J., Mitchell, J., Parker, S., Morelock, S., & Timperi, R. (1986). Maternal marijuana use and neonatal outcome: Uncertainty posed by self-reports. *American Journal of Public Health, 76*, 667-669.

Hoerlin, Bettina Yaffe, Ph.D. (1989, Spring). *Connecting: Challenges in Health and Human Services in the Philadelphia Region.* A Study Sponsored by the Pew Charitable Trusts.

Howard, J., Beckwith, L., Rodning, C., & Kropenske, V. (1989). The development of young children of substance-abusing parents: Insights from seven years of intervention and research. *Zero to Three, 9*, 8-12.

Kagan, S.L., Powell, D.R., Weissbourd, B., & Zigler, E.F. (1987). *America's family support programs.* New Haven: Yale University Press.

Lief, N.R. (1985). The drug user as parent. *The International Journal of Addictions, 20*, 63-97.

McLellan, T., Luborsky, L., Cacciola, J., Griffith, J., Evans, F., Barr, H., & O'Brien, C. (1985). New data from the Addiction Severity Index: Reliability and validity in three centers. *Journal of Nervous and Mental Disease, 173,* 412-423.

Mullins, C.L., & Gazaway, P.M., III (1985). Alcohol and drug use in pregnancy: A case for management. *MMJ, 34* (10), 991-996.

Philadelphia Perinatal Society, Philadelphia Department of Public Health. (1989). One thousand babies: Philadelphia, 1989. Paper presented at a Seminar on The Effects of Substance Abuse on Fetal and Newborn Development, Temple Medical School, Philadelphia.

Regan, D.O., Ehrlich, S.M., & Finnegan, L. (1987). Infants of drug addicts: At risk for child abuse, neglect, and placement in foster care. *Neurotoxicology and Teratology, 9*, 315-319.

Schorr, L.B., with Schorr, D. (1988). *Within Our Reach: Breaking the Cycle of Disadvantage*. New York: Anchor Press/Doubleday.

Shandler, I.W., & Shipley, T.E. (1987). New focus for an old problem: Philadelphia's response to homelessness: *Alcohol Health and Research World, 11*, 54-56.

State of New Jersey Commission of Investigation, (1989). *Cocaine*. Trenton, New Jersey.

Sullivan, P.A., & Damrosch, S.P. (1987). *The Homeless in Contemporary Society*. Newbury Park: Sage Publications.

Weston, D.R., Ivins, B., Zuckerman, B., Jones, C., & Lopez, R. (1989). Drug exposed babies: Research and clinical issues. *Zero to Three, 9*, 1-7.

Wiegand, G. (November 27, 1988). Cocaine invades a woman's world. *The Philadelphia Inquirer*, p. E7.

Implementation of Rehabilitation Program for Dually Diagnosed Homeless

Laura Blankertz, PhD
Kalma Kartell White, MEd

Comprehensive Rehabilitation Services for Dually Diagnosed Homeless Persons is dedicated to working with undomiciled adults who have co-occurring mental health and substance abuse problems. The major goal of this Project is to provide comprehensive services which focus on the reduction/elimination of alcohol and other drug abuse, the improvement of mental health functioning, and the provision of opportunities for client acquisition of the skills and supports necessary to develop economic and social self-sufficiency. This project differs from the other nine NIAAA Homeless Demonstration Projects both in its target population and in the intensive nature of the rehabilitation services that it provides. Many of these services, especially the residential units and those provided by other programs within Horizon House, utilize the philosophy and techniques of psychosocial rehabilitation; a client driven process emphasizing client empowerment. Psychosocial rehabilitation focuses on teaching individuals the specific social, residential, vocational and educational skills they need to meet their chosen rehabilitation goal. Strong client-provider relationships are established, which motivate clients to achieve their goals, stabilize their lives and help them develop the decision-making skills necessary to control their lives (Cnaan, Blankertz, Messinger and Gardner, 1988).

To deliver this level of services, the project is structured to provide residential placement and rehabilitation for 53 individuals at any one time. Case managers concomitantly work with individuals

Laura Blankertz and Kalma Kartell White are affiliated with Horizon House, 120 South 30th Street, Philadelphia, PA 19104.

149

on the street and in other shelters to "engage" them to come into the project; with those that have "graduated" from the program but still need monitoring and personal support; and with those that have left or have been asked to leave the project.

DESCRIPTION OF TARGET POPULATION

The purpose of the project is to work intensively in a holistic fashion with dually diagnosed homeless individuals so that all of the multiple problems which prevent them from attaining independent living can be simultaneously addressed.

In developing its program format, the project has had to be innovative and flexible. It is only in the last several years that dually diagnosed individuals have become a recognized subpopulation of the homeless (Barrow et al., 1986; Schutt and Garrett, 1988; Koegel and Burnham, in press; Dennis, 1987). Services targeted for this group are also lacking. Individuals with dual problems have often fallen between the cracks between the mental health and substance abuse service systems. Often domiciled, dually diagnosed individuals are refused admittance to programs in both the mental health and substance abuse systems. Their usage of psychotropic medications often prevents admittance into programs in the drug and alcohol system which require abstinence from all mood-altering drugs. Their use and/or abuse of controlled substances denies them entrance into mental health programs. The disruptive, non-compliant behavior of some of these individuals may additionally bar them from programs in either system (Hellerstein and Meeham, 1987; Pinsker, 1983). If they are served in one system, according to the system's normal treatment pattern, the concurrent disorder is usually ignored and there is often a high dropout/morbidity rate among them (McClellan et al., 1988; Safer, 1987; Pinsker, 1983). Unfortunately, for many dually diagnosed homeless individuals, the legal system has become the service provider of last resort (Schutt and Garrett, 1988; Koegel and Burnham, in press).

Literature on the treatment and rehabilitation of individuals with dual problems is scarce and focuses on domiciled dually diagnosed clients. While it suggests that both disorders must be treated simultaneously (Safer, 1987; Hellerstein and Meeham, 1987; Ridgely et al., 1987), there are very few program descriptions for this population and even less documentation of outcomes. The few descriptions that do exist (and these are found primarily in the mental health literature) focus on the utilization of groups to develop motivation in individuals with mental health problems to directly work on their substance abuse. These groups often have two group leaders, one from each field, or leaders that are cross-trained (Kofoed and Keys, 1988; Hellerstein and Meehan, 1987).

A factor that has made program development more difficult is the unknown dimensions of this population. Little is known about the variations related to different types of dual disorder interrelationships, different sociodemographic characteristics, and subsequent differing service needs.

It has been suggested that there are subgroups based upon the different interrelationships of the mental health and substance abuse disorders (Osher, 1988; White and White, forthcoming). However, no typologies have been empirically validated. Heterogeneity is increased by the fact that each type of mental disability may evidence differing behavior when combined with different substances (Galanter and Castaneda, 1988).

Koegal and Burnham have found dually diagnosed homeless in Los Angeles to be similar to long-term mentally disabled homeless with respect to some of their sociodemographic characteristics; similar to alcoholic homeless on other characteristics; and unique in others.

What is completely unknown about dually diagnosed individuals is their service profile or their service needs. How much engagement, structure and limit-setting do they need? Do they need a long period of engagement similar to the longterm mentally disabled homeless, or do they need structured limits similar to the substance-abusing homeless? Are they able or willing to participate in programs that make structured demands and are time-limited, similar to episodically homeless young adults, or are they unwilling or at functional levels that do not permit them to tolerate structured demands similar to deinstitutionalized long-term "street people?" The vast heterogeneity of this target group suggests that service needs will vary according to the intensity of their mental disabilities, their substance of choice, and their emotional and social background. To meet such varying needs, the Horizon House project has established a rehabilitation/service program which is flexible and individualized.

DESCRIPTION OF PROGRAM ELEMENTS

Residential Alternatives

There are three residential sites within which the program takes place. These are funded by different components of the human service system in Philadelphia, a situation which has also created linkages for the project. These sites are a large group home which has 28 beds; 15 board and care slots in the homes of approved and trained providers; and 10 supported independent housing units. For the most part, these three alternatives represent a continuum of residential rehabilitation. When individuals first enter the program, they come directly to the large group home. Here their dual problems are assessed, they choose individual rehabilitation goals, and they are immediately linked with entitlements and needed substance abuse treatment, as well as mental health and physical health care. As individuals become adjusted to the program, they are linked with the appropriate day programs and problem-oriented educational/support groups both on- and off-site. Once a client has demonstrated sufficient mastery of daily living skills and has made significant strides towards stabilizing his/her mental health problems and attaining abstinence, he/she can then move on to either the board and care or independent living situations. Designated for clients of different functional levels, these latter residences provide less structure and supports than the large group house although there is a case manager on call at all times.

Service Components

There are four interlocking components of the program, all working within the structure of psychosocial rehabilitation, with its emphasis on client choice and client empowerment. These four subcomponents are outreach/engagement; initial assessments and linkages; individual rehabilitation and service planning; residential groups and day programs. In all of these, the relationship of the

case manager with the client is the vital, underlying strand, responsible for activating and integrating the components.

Outreach/Engagement

Case managers serve as outreach workers and go to the streets or
shelters on a regular basis. "Engagement" refers to the process of
establishing trust and rapport with clients. The element of engagement is vital to developing an effective relationship between the
case manager and clients with the intent of helping to develop the
environmental resources and client skills necessary to deal with
their dual issues.

The engagement process can take a very long period of time
(Rog, 1987; Barrow and Lovell, 1982). Long-term homeless individuals have developed their own lifestyle with values and customs
adaptive to protecting themselves and maintaining self esteem
(Snow, 1988). Many have a strong desire for autonomy and privacy. They also display suspicion and hostility towards others, particularly toward service providers with whom they often have had
negative experiences. Although these characteristics have been described as "disaffiliation" (Bahr, 1970; Rossi et al., 1986; Bach-
rach, 1984), they also serve a positive or adaptive function in a
lifestyle often fraught with danger.

Because of the constant stress of living on the streets and the
distortions related to mental disability and substance abuse, the
worlds of these homeless individuals can appear to be chaotic and
bizarre. Outreach/engagement workers try to become an accepted
part of the individual's world. Contacts by project staff are initially
very low key, respectful, and cautious. The workers let the clients
set the length and nature of the initial interchanges. Workers offer
immediate concrete services to the individual (e.g., telling them
where meals are; offering to help them get benefits; making them
aware of the availability of shelter). Sometimes the worker's goal
may simply be to communicate that a helper will be back again.
Gradually, over a period of time, the potential clients come to accept the worker, and to interact with them on a positive basis. It is
only later, after this connection has been made, that the worker will
try to "bring in" the client. This process can take many months.

Horizon House case managers have been on targeted outreach since July 1988. They have made a total of 566 contacts with homeless persons and have identified 75 individuals as being potentially dually diagnosed. Outreach statistics reveal that those identified as potentially dually diagnosed are predominantly black (71%), male (83%), and middle-aged (60% are between the ages of 36 and 64).

Initial Assessment and Linkages with Basic Services and Entitlements

When clients enter the project, one of the first activities undertaken on their behalf by case managers is to link clients with financial entitlements (SSI and DPA). Of the 34 clients case managed so far, only 5 had to have the process initiated by the case manager. Although it may take a while for case managers to attain the information, most of the clients have been previously linked financially to a service system. Also, all clients receive basic mental and physical health assessments to ensure that they are linked with the appropriate immediate health care.

Second, the case managers continue to assess clients to determine if they are indeed dually diagnosed. Because of the lack of a consistent definition in the field of dual diagnosis, the project has developed its own working definition. The establishment of such a definition is necessary if an assessment is to take place. For the purpose of the Horizon House project, an individual is to be considered dually diagnosed if he or she has severe, persistent mental health problems (i.e., medically identified as schizophrenia, schixophreneiform disorder, delusional disorder, schizoaffective disorders, mood disorders, and borderline personality disorders) and there is continued use of psychoactive substances, despite the existence of a persistent or recurrent social, occupational, or physical problem that is caused or exacerbated by the use of these substances. This definition has been chosen to reflect the fact that some persons with mental health disorders may be highly sensitive to the use of small amounts of psychoactive substances (Ridgely, Osher, Goldman and Talbott, 1987).

Assessment regarding whether an individual can be labelled as dually diagnosed can be a lengthy process. It can be very difficult to determine the exact dimensions of the two presenting problems because they may mutually exacerbate and mimic each other in some of their symptoms (Pinsker, 1987; Galanter and Castaneda, 1988). There are two questions that drive the assessment process. First, are there in actuality two co-existing disorders (or do the behaviors related to one disorder present as symptoms of the second)? A major concern of the project staff is a clear determination as to whether there is an actual major mental health condition present. Providing psychotropic medication when it is not needed can not only physically harm the client, but can also enable that individual to continue substance abuse. Second, which is the primary and which is the secondary disorder? (Or which is the basic disorder and which is the derivative?) For example, major depression that has preceded alcoholism is treated differently from the depression that often accompanies alcoholism and its withdrawal; drug induced psychosis requires different interventions from that which is needed to address substance use/abuse pursued to reduce the effects of a primary psychosis. Determining the answers to these questions is vital for selecting the appropriate rehabilitation interventions to maximize the outcome. To assure maximum accuracy, the case manager works closely with the psychiatrists, substance abuse service providers and residential staff to obtain information on the dual problems. Complete psychosocial histories as well as clinical observations and client self-report are valuable tools. This information is constantly reevaluated at case conference.

Individual Rehabilitation and Service Planning

Project programming individualizes and superimposes principles of the Therapeutic Community on a low demand residence format. This structure gives maximum flexibility to meet the varying needs of this heterogeneous homeless subpopulation for engagement, structure, and limit-setting.

Many dually diagnosed individuals can not tolerate a highly structured, restrictive environment, such as a traditional therapeutic community, after living on the streets. They are not willing to relinquish their sense of self-determination (autonomy) and freedom which have been major sources of self-esteem and have given them the strength to survive (Baxter and Hopper, 1982). Many, because of their previous life experiences or because of their mental health status, are not willing or able to handle a high level of demand in many areas simultaneously. In addition, many of the dually diagnosed long-term homeless are not willing to strive for immediate abstinence. These individuals do not have a commitment to abstinence because either they are addicted, substance abuse is an integral part of their lifestyle and values, or substance abuse has been a means of avoiding the harsh reality of life on the streets. (Some, indeed, have been using substances to "self-medicate" their mental health issues.) Faced with an environment with structured rigid rules and required compliance, many will leave. (This has also been observed for domiciled dually diagnosed individuals.)

In order to truly serve the targeted population and not just "cream" off a small percentage of the most able and motivated clients, Horizon House has adopted the format of a low demand residence for the initial stage of its project, the large group home. A "Low Demand Residence" (LDR) is a type of program available for the homeless in both the mental health and substance abuse service systems of Philadelphia. Initially, the LDR makes few demands on its residents. As individuals adjust to life off the streets, the program adjusts and heightens its expectations of individuals.

In addition, the project has superimposed upon this LDR format the structure of an individualized, client-driven adaptation of the Therapeutic Community approach and principles. This is operationalized by a "contract-driven" system. At the point of entry into the program, the client assumes the responsibility of "tenancy" and its accompanying rules which are written in the form of an initial contract. If the client is a person who needs structure and limits and violates the rules of the residence, which include a curfew and the prohibition of substance usage on the premises, then a contingency contract is developed which spells out consequences, both positive and negative, and carefully describes the conditions to be fulfilled by both staff and client. The individualization of this contract is compatible with the psychosocial rehabilitation process, which features an individualized rehabilitation plan developed by residential staff with the client and an individualized service plan, developed by the case manager. Both plans reflect the values, goals and choices of the client. There is some indication from literature in the field (Pinsker, 1983) that unless the dually diagnosed individual freely chooses to embark on a rehabilitation process, that rehabilitation will not be effective. The individual rehabilitation plan includes specific goals chosen by the client. These goals vary from individual to individual, depending upon interest, motivation, abilities and previous life histories. Rehabilitation plans also outline the specific skills clients need to learn to reach their goals. Case managers, via the individual service plan, delineate the specific resources, including mental health care and substance abuse rehabilitation, that are needed to help improve the quality of life for clients. The purpose of these three rehabilitative tools (the service plan, the rehabilitation plan, and the contract) is to facilitate work with the client to both make choices and "own" the choices they make, accepting the responsibility for failures as well as successes. Given the low self esteem of many of these individuals, staff work to have the contracts and the rehabilitation plans reflect aims and goals that can be achieved and thus bring successes. Case managers and residential counselors, through the working relationship, continuously encourage clients to choose rehabilitation goals and activities that focus on attaining abstinence and stabilizing mental health.

The working relationship developed between the client and case manager/residential counselor is a powerful means of motivating clients to achieve their rehabilitation goals, to meet their contract obligations and to help them attain an awareness of the consequences of their substance abuse. If the client continually violates contracts or the rules of the residence (such as using contraband drugs on the premises), that individual's residency in the program will be terminated. However, he or she will not be dropped from the project. The case manager will continue to work with the client to find shelter, although perhaps not in the same circumstances as the facility he or she has just left. The case manager will also work to maintain the relationship with the client, continuing to treat that individual with dignity and respect but without enabling substance abuse or manipulative behavior. Programmatic failure or other crises often serve as growth experiences. Having to face the consequences of problematic behavior, the client can often, with continued case management support, begin to make different, more positive choices. To date, two of the seven clients who have left the program are ready to re-enter.

Day Programs and Psychoeducational and Self-Help Groups

In addition to working on skills and resource acquisition as outlined in individual residential rehabilitation and case management service plans, clients attend individual day programs and groups which deal with dual problem issues. Day programs are chosen to meet the specific needs of the client. Although there are a variety of programs available within the Horizon House organization, case managers can and do link clients to programs throughout the city. Currently, clients are attending partial hospital day programs oriented to work on dual problems, drug and alcohol outpatient services, and a clubhouse program that focuses on mental health concerns.

The groups include both psychoeducational groups run either by residential staff or case managers and self help groups run by recovering dually diagnosed individuals. The psychoeducation groups focus on engagement into the group; informational discussions during which clients collectively recognize and talk about the negative impact of substance abuse on their mental health; and promotion of positive group support for participants who are struggling to acknowledge their substance abuse and participants who are working towards abstinence. The self help groups include on-site and off-site Double Trouble, Narcotics Anonymous and Alcohol Anonymous meetings.

SYSTEM LINKAGES

To facilitate successful program implementation, the project has created linkages with other agencies, organizations and providers in the city. Creation of these linkages has been necessitated because the two different systems traditionally responsible for mental health and substance abuse in Philadelphia have different funding streams and separate organizational mechanisms. Several methods have been used to develop cooperation and formalized relationships.

First, the project has created a task force which brings together in quarterly meetings all agencies and organizations that are involved with the NIAAA Community Demonstration Project in any way. Secondly, the project director attends all task forces and citywide committees that deal with homelessness issues. Philadelphia has no formal structure to coordinate all of the public, not-for-profit, and religious organizations that are, nevertheless, key elements in the human service system. Membership on overlapping committees is the best way to ensure coordination, communication and cooperation. Thirdly, the project has developed special working agreements with individual providers and agencies for specialized services for dually diagnosed clients. Fourth, the case managers make direct contacts as they work across agencies to attain the necessary resources to meet the needs of the clients. As a result of these linkages, it is anticipated that the provider community will become more informed regarding dual diagnosis topics of concern, existing services will be maximally accessed, and service deficits for this sub-population will be identified. The fifth strategy has been to include providers of mental health/substance abuse and other services to the homeless in project training on dual diagnostic issues.

As a result of these linkage activities, coordinated outreach to dually diagnosed homeless persons has increased in the city; service providers have become aware of the complexity and length of time needed to correctly assess a homeless individual as "dually diagnosed," and specific services have been attained for the clients including detoxification, health care programs and day programming slots.

EVALUATION

Evaluation has been an integral part of the project from its inception. The Project is using a quasi-experimental research design, with one nonequivalent comparison group (another residential program for dually diagnosed homeless operated by an agency whose emphasis is primarily on drug and alcohol rehabilitation), and one nonequivalent control group, i.e., a waiting list of those individuals for the two programs. Three repeated measures (administered every six months) are used to record changes in these three groups, the

Addiction Severity Index, a homeless functional assessment, and Rosenberg's Self Esteem Index. Extensive data bases have been created, which track the characteristics, services received and outcomes of individual clients. Because so little is known about this subpopulation of the homeless, the client data bases have an extensive personal history and background section. Two research assistants are on site full-time because they too have found it necessary to establish a trusting work relationship with the clients if they are to gather valid reliable information.

In addition, qualitative data on the reactions of the staff and clients to the project is gathered on an outgoing basis. During the first year, the residential staff, as well as the case managers, struggled with "burnout," as they worked with clients who were especially manipulative and resistant. (As explained below, these clients represent some of the most difficult in the city, "dumped" on the project when it opened.) Staff have also experienced the stresses inherent in group formation, as they, individuals with backgrounds in two different service systems (mental health and substance abuse) struggled to merge themselves into one tight unit that communicated succinctly with respect to client needs.

BARRIERS TO IMPLEMENTATION

One significant barrier which the project faced in the first year was the delay in the opening of the 28-bed group home, which is the first stage and assessment center for the project. Delays were caused by the lack of total control over the facility (which Horizon House was compelled to rent) and its renovations. Within the city of Philadelphia, there is a severe shortage of buildings large enough to contain a group home that meet certain crucial specifications: i.e., location in areas indigenous to the homeless; appropriate zoning; and no overwhelming community opposition. Many long-term homeless people, create for themselves a "home," which constitutes a territory within a set geographic area such as a certain neighborhood or city sector. They often refuse to leave this "home" area. Unfortunately, large buildings that are in the physical area where many of the homeless are to be found and that are appropriately zoned are hard to find. After a fruitless canvas of the major target areas, no buildings for purchase could be found and the agency finally rented a building. However, by the terms of the lease, the building owner was to be in charge of the renovations. However, he did not complete the physical work on schedule; nor did he file the appropriate paperwork for licensure. Horizon House was forced to intervene legally and additionally worked with a specially appointed delegate of the city to get the licensure paperwork through the appropriate channels as quickly as possible.

A second barrier was the inability of the project to immediately access the 15 board and care home slots committed to the project by the Philadelphia Office of Services to Homeless Adults (OSHA) at the time of the grant application. Between the time the grant was written and awarded, there was a change in top leadership at OSHA. Horizon House had to reinitiate the entire process of presenting the project, gaining approval, and creating protocols.

A third barrier has been the general lack of knowledge of dual diagnosis in the Philadelphia human service system. This deficit has affected the project in several significant ways. First, the project has had to educate the community, including agency administrators and providers, as to the nature and characteristics of dual diagnosis. It was discovered that leaders within the mental health and drug and alcohol systems had different definitions of this subpopulation, and did not seem to be aware of the complexity of the assessment process. The project has spent time at the various task force meetings explaining the nature of dual diagnosis and has also offered training to the community at large on the characteristics of the interventions for this subpopulation.

Because of this lack of knowledge, many provider agencies often refer inappropriate candidates to the project. Many of these people are "heavy users" of the mental health system who have not been successfully placed elsewhere. To avoid being the repository for "system dumpees," the project spent much time discussing the nature of dual diagnosis with providers; carefully assessing these referrals; and, if they were inappropriate, creating linkages so that they could be served elsewhere.

Second, the project has faced a lack of appropriate services in the community. For example, there are few day and residential programs for dually diagnosed, few detoxification facilities, and few clean and sober dedicated housing units. The project has been working to create linkages as a base from which such services can be developed.

Third, because dual problem clients have not been recognized as such until recently and some exhibit behavior which is difficult for many practitioners to manage, the case managers and residential staff needed specialized training. This training was also opened to other providers in the community. It included information on substance abuse and mental health, drug interactions, the mental health and substance abuse service systems, contract contingency training, and rehabilitation approaches including twelve-step, Therapeutic Community, and the psychosocial model.

CONCLUSION

Despite some initial barriers, the Horizon House project has been able to make substantial progress in its first year of working with this challenging and service resistant subpopulation of the homeless. Project staff have been able to make the necessary linkages and formalized agreements to attain and develop needed resources for clients. A program format has been created which is flexibly individualized to meet the specific combination of engagement, structure and limits needed by each dually diagnosed client. Intensive case management has provided a strong underlying foundation, creating a provider-client relationship which can be used to motivate and support abstinence and help a client grow towards making decisions that take into account the consequences of his or her actions. An extensive evaluation data base has been developed which will not only measure program implementation but also provide researchers and providers with valuable insights into the nature of dual diagnosis and the environmental factors which impact upon it.

As the project continues to gain momentum and the provider community becomes more cognizant of dual diagnosis issues, it is expected that the project will have permanent impact on the service system by forming a permanent task force on dual diagnosis which will assess the array of services available and advocate for changes, such as specialized sober housing and specialized detoxification. A coordinated, comprehensive approach is critically needed to offer the needed services for these multiple problem individuals to gain the skills and supports to attain productive independence living.

BIBLIOGRAPHY

Bahr, H.M. (1970) *Disaffiliated Man: Essays and Bibliography on Homelessness*. University of Toronto Press.

Barrow, S., Stuening, E., Plapinger, J., Hemlamm, F. and Lovell, A. (1986). *Effectiveness of Services for the Mentally Ill Homeless*. New York State Psychiatric Institute.

Barrow, S., and Lovell, A. (1982) *Evaluation of Project Reachout, 1981-82*. New York State Psychiatric Institute.

Cnaan, R., Blankertz, L., Messinger, K., and Gardner, J. (1988) "Psychosocial rehabilitation: Toward a definition" *Psychosocial Rehabilitation Journal, 11* (4), pp. 68-78.

Dennis, D.L. (1987). *Research Methodologies Concerning Homeless Persons with Serious Mental Illness and or Substance Abuse Disorders*. NIMH.

Galanter, M. and Castaneda, R. (1988) "Substance abuse among general psychiatric patients: Place of presentation, diagnosis and treatment" *American J. Drug Alcohol Abuse, 14* (2), pp 211-235.

Hellerstein, D. and Meehan, B. (1987). "Outpatient group therapy for schizophrenic substance abusers" *American J. of Psychiatry, 144* (10).

Koegel P., Burnham, M.A. and Farr, R.K. (in press). *Archives of General Psychiatry*.

Kofoed, L. and Keys, A. (1988). "Using group therapy to persuade dual diagnosis patients to seek substance abuse treatment." *Hospital and Community Psychiatry, 39* (11).

McLellan, A.T., Luborsky, L. and Woods, G. et al. (1983). *Archives of General Psychiatry 40*, pp. 620-22.

Osher, F. (1988) Conference Proceedings. CSP Conference on Demonstration Grants for Young Adults with Mental Illness and Substance Abuse Problems. Rockville, Md.

Pinsker, H. (1983). "Addicted patients in hospital psychiatric units" *Psychiatric Annals, 13* (8).

Ridgely, M. S. Osher, F.C. and Talbott, J.A. (1987). *Chronic Mentally Ill Young Adults with Substance Abuse Problems: Treatment and Training Issues*. University of Maryland.

Rossi, P., Wright, J., Fisher, B., and Willis, G. (1987) "The urban homeless: Estimating composition and size" *Science 235* (3), pp. 1336-41.

Rog, D.J. (1988) *Engaging Homeless Persons with Mental Illness into Treatment*. Alexandria, Va. National Mental Health Association.

Safer, D. (1987) "Substance abuse by young adult chronic patients" *Hospital and Community Psychiatry, 38* (5).

Schutt, R. and Garrett, G. (1988). "Social background, residential experience and health problems of the homeless. *Psychosocial Rehabilitation Journal, 12* (3).

White, K. and White, D. "Dual mental health and substance use problems: A model of four subtypes" forthcoming, *Psychosocial Rehabilitation Journal.*